TECHNIQUES
IN
ADULT
CRICOTHYROID MEMBRANE
EMERGENCY ULTRASOUND
LOCALIZATION

TECHNIQUES
IN
ADULT
CRICOTHYROID MEMBRANE
EMERGENCY ULTRASOUND
LOCALIZATION

Authored by

Jacob-Sung Sik Keum D.O. Author
Emergency Medicine Physician
Orchard Hospital
Gridley, California
Community Hospital Huntington Park
Huntington Park, California

Edited by

Tomoko Ikuine M.D. Chief Editor
Senior Resident Physician, Internal Medicine
Department of Medicine
St John's Episcopal Hospital Far Rockaway, New York

Scott Ladd D.O., M.H.S. Associate Chief Editor
Attending Physician, Hospital Medicine
Orchard Hospital, Gridley, California
The Johns Hopkins Bloomberg School of Public Health

Demetrius Christoforatos M.D. Consultant Editor
Attending Physician in Anesthesiology
Northeastern Eye Institute Scranton, Pennsylvania

William Kurzbuch M.D. Research Editor
Veteran of United States Navy
Keum Biomedical Sciences Inc Sheridan, Wyoming

Michael Njoku R.N. Research Editor
Keum Biomedical Sciences Inc   Sheridan, Wyoming

Jacob-Sung Sik Keum DO
with Keum Biomedical Sciences Inc Publishing.

Jacob-Sung Sik Keum DO with
Keum Biomedical Sciences Inc Publishing
Sheridan, Wyoming, United States of America

The Publishing Unit is an independent division of
Keum Biomedical Sciences Inc.
It has the mission to develop new ideas in medicine and
surgery with the goal of advancing medical education,
research and development globally.

First Publication 2021

Printed in the United States of America
by Amazon Kindle Direct Publishing in authorized formats.

Techniques in Adult Cricothyroid Membrane Emergency
Ultrasound Localization authored by
Jacob-Sung S. Keum,
and edited by
Tomoko Ikuine, Scott Ladd,
Demetrius Christoforatos,
William Kurzbuch, Michael Njoku.
Includes index.
Copyright © 2021 by Jacob-Sung S. Keum D.O.
Library of Congress Control Number: 2021901138
ISBN-13 978-1-7365179-1-8 (Hardback)
ISBN-13 978-1-7365179-0-1 (Paperback)

I. Keum, Jacob-Sung S., 1969- , author.
II. Ikuine, Tomoko, chief editor.
III. Ladd, Scott, associate editor.
IV. Kurzbuch, William, research editor.
V. Christoforatos, Demetrius, consulting editor.
VI. Njoku, Michael, research editor.

ISBN-13 978-1-7365179-0-1 (paperback)

ISBN 978-1-7365179-0-1

90000>

9 781736 517901

Dedication

I want to give thanks to my family, friends and colleagues for supporting me with these new ideas.

The development of this book occurred before and during the COVID-19 pandemic. Thank you to all our healthcare Workers.

I want to give special thanks to:

Doctors Tomoko Ikuine, Scott Ladd, William Kurzbuch, Demetrius Christoforatos, and Nurse Researcher Michael Njoku for your valuable contributions in the completion of this book.

Also I want to give my appreciation to all the administration and staff at The Eastern Long Island Hospital in Greenport, New York including special mention to Doctors Lawrence Schiff ER Director and Kai Sturmann Associate Director for all their support.

I also want to mention the tremendous support i received from my ER nursing staff at the Orchard Hospital from Elizabeth Brown, Dianne Kieffer, Aimee Merchant, Krystal Schumaker, Linda Sundberg, Fidel Castro, Christy Sewell, Kimberly McReynolds, Gail Shimmin, Rhonda Harvey, Sonya Ramirez, Denise Lincoln, Seth Marston, Shilow Beltran, Elizabeth Rutter-James, Katherine Townsend, Jennifer Cabrera, Aminah Khan, Lori Clark, ER clerks Cari Edgerton, Martha James, and all other ancillary staff. Furthermore, i want to give my sincere appreciation to the entire Orchard Hospital administration CEO Steve Stark, Patricia Stahlberg medical staff, John Helvey CIO, Patricia Taverner IT and to all my ER physician colleagues Lucy Douglass, Greg Ishimoto, Cynthia Cellucci, Jeremy Martinez, Richard Kaut, Kevin Maxwell, Jack C. Lane, Salah Sherif, Thomas Wendel, and all our Hospitalist team.

I want to make special mention to Doctors Kohji Uzawa, Joho Tokumine, Okano and their team at Kyorin University School of Medicine in Tokyo, Japan and Doctor Mikael Haggstrom for their generosity in giving us their permission to use photographs from their respective publications.

To all our readers, We hope the knowledge contained in this book can help you take care of your patients in critical hours to the next level of excellence.

INTRODUCTION

My name is Jacob-Sung Sik Keum D.O.
I am a General Practice Osteopathic Physician practicing
Emergency Medicine in Gridley and in Los Angeles California.

For all those readers from outside of the United States,
I wanted to clarify one thing: Since 1965, the US Osteopathic
Physicians attained full medical and surgical practice rights in
the United States. Since that time all the D.O. (Doctor of
Osteopathic Medicine) degree holders in the United States of
America have the same and equal physician practice privileges
like M.D. (Medical Doctor) in all US territory.
And, Doctors of Osteopathic Medicine are represented in all
medical and surgical specialties.

I have decided to write this book on ultrasound guided
localization of the cricothyroid membrane back in 2018.

We have heard about people using a pen to puncture the neck
during a severe choking event to save someone's life. For the
general public, this simple mechanical action of puncturing
someone's neck with a sharp object to alleviate life threatening
choking events can be seen as a very simple act.

From the medical practitioners' perspective, the
cricothyroidotomy (the emergency surgical procedure for
management of airway obstruction) is an uncommon procedure
practiced very rarely. (42)

And, the most challenging part of this life saving procedure is the <u>precise localization of the cricothyroid membrane</u>.

This localization process requires more than a solid theoretical knowledge of the neck anatomy. (45) There are many important structures proximal to the cricothyroid membrane: from upper alimentary tract, large blood vessels, nerves, the thyroid gland, the vocal cord and trachea among others.

It is not surprising to hear often Emergency Room stories in which the vocal cord was permanently damaged during a cricothyroidotomy due to errors in the manual anatomical identification during this important procedure leading to actual failure to complete the procedure.

In this book, we are going to present new ways to approach the localization of cricothyroid membrane by building up our basic knowledge of anatomy and ultrasound skills in the neck region.

With patience and practice we will acquire the ability to systematically Identify the cricothyroid membrane for the cricothyroidotomy using all visual, tactile and ultrasound modalities.

OBJECTIVES

The traditional cricothyroidotomy is a procedure based on anatomical estimation. Foremost, the operating surgeon must identify the precise location of the cricothyroid membrane. The successful performance of the cricothyroidotomy is directly proportional to the operator's experience and his or her knowledge of anatomy of the cricothyroid membrane and the neck region.

This book was written with the main objective to teach all healthcare professionals working in Critical Medicine, Emergency Medicine, Hospital Medicine, Trauma Surgery including all prehospital providers and those first responders practicing in the most remote and rural areas the basic and ultrasound guided anatomy of the adult cricothyroid membrane and its ultrasound guided localization in an adult patients (including pediatric patients older than 11 years) and in a systematic manner with ultrasound in preparation of performing cricothyroidotomy in cases of emergent upper airway obstruction.

By using, a systematic ultrasound scanning protocol to correctly identify the cricothyroid membrane, the operating surgeon can concentrate on the actual procedure instead of approximating the exact location where The first incision of cricothyrotomy should be made.

In addition, the rapid systematic ultrasound scanning can assist in early detection of significant laryngeal injury in trauma scenarios as an added advantage in its utilization. (63)

Firstly, this book will review the key anatomical landmarks of cricothyroid membrane visually in all different axis, then it will present the ultrasound guided anatomy of these structures using easily recalled mnemonics.

Finally, we will study five ultrasound-guided localization techniques created from my own personal scanning experience. And, we will also review a well known ultrasound confirmation technique: the paperclip shadow confirmation technique.

This book is not a procedural atlas providing instructions on how to perform the surgical, percutaneous or needle cricothyroidotomy because there are many publications available for that purpose.

But what is learned from the ultrasound-guided localization of pertinent anatomy can open multiple possibilities on how the actual procedures can be improved in its performance.

The true mastery is not about knowing one way to do a task but rather the ability to think outside of the box and be intellectually flexible to achieve the same goal using different techniques.

This book will give you a solid foundation on the practical anatomical knowledge needed to become a skillful airway surgeon.

CONTENTS

The book is structured into two main sections.

The first section has four chapters which gives the operating surgeon brief background information on indications of cricothyroidotomy and the necessary equipment for scanning.

We will also briefly review the required basic ultrasound scan settings.

Finally, this section includes the visualization of the anatomical landmarks in different orientations to serve as a review and the entire chapter on ultrasound correlations with easily recalled mnemonic terminologies that I developed to aid in remembering these important sonographic landmarks.

The second section of the book comprises of two chapters; Chapter 5 will go over the TSTS and 5s scanning protocols. (These are more comprehensive scanning protocols). They were created to review and to get the airway surgeon familiarized with all the important anatomical landmarks under ultrasound guidance.

Chapter 6 will go over the fastest way to localize the cricothyroid membrane including a second variant of the protocol which includes an ultrasonographic view designed for the actual procedural view.

It will touch upon the paperclip shadow confirmation technique which can be utilized to correlate the relationship between the skin level to visual information from the structures seen in the scanned ultrasound images.

All ultrasound images in this book were obtained from my own personal scanning sessions using following diagnostic ultrasound scanners from their respective makers:

> Chison Q9 made by Chison
> C3 multi-use wireless probe by Clarius
> Site Rite Vision Ultrasound System by Bard

Finally, after using different scanners from different makers, the ultrasound localization techniques presented in this book can be easily applied by all practitioners with any properly functioning diagnostic ultrasound scanner. This is assuming proper time is devoted to studying these techniques in order to acquire a solid knowledge of all important anatomical structures in the neck region so during those critical clinical encounters when a surgical airway is needed then you can be sufficiently prepared to perform the cricothyroidotomy or tracheostomy with greater confidence.

Contents

Chapter 1

**The ultrasound guided localization
the cricothyroid membrane
in surgical, percutaneous or
needle Cricothyroidotomy. <u>Why</u>?**

The classic cricothyroidotomy is an emergency surgical
procedure based mainly on manual palpation of the
cricothyroid membrane.
It is preferred over tracheotomy because of its much lower
incidence of complications including subglottic stenosis.
(54)(55)(61)
When we say that this is a manual palpation, it refers to the
tactile examination of the neck region leading to a operator's
estimation about the exact location of the cricothyroid
membrane or CTM.

So, It is strictly an <u>operator-dependent procedure</u>.

The accuracy of the procedure is directly dependent on
the past experience of the operating surgeon, and his or her
knowledge of the anatomy of the neck region.

In time sensitive situations, traumatologist have used the four closed finger hand methodology to locate the cricothyroid membrane. (55)

This Manual Localization Method consists of the Airway Surgeon using his or her dominant hand to estimate the correct position of the cricothyroid membrane by using the hand size width as the distance from the suprasternal notch to the cricothyroid membrane location. This book will discuss the details of this particular localization method.

THE LARYNGEAL HANDSHAKE METHOD

This is another palpatory technique which can be used quickly to Identify the thyroid cartilage and cricothyroid membrane. Use your dominant hand and grasp the thyroid cartilage in the sagittal or lateral axis.

This technique assumes the superior part of thyroid cartilage is held in between the thumb and the index finger and if the palpation is correct, then you may be able to gently rock the thyroid cartilage in a lateral motion. If you have correctly identified the thyroid cartilage, the gentle side by side motion will produce a very unique clicking sound. This is the sound made by thyroid cartilage rocking motion.

The logic of this technique is if you can correctly identify the thyroid cartilage then with a greater certainty you will locate the cricothyroid membrane by simply sliding inferiorly along the anterior walls of the thyroid cartilage until your fingers reach the superior border of the cricothyroid membrane. (56)

THE LARYNGEAL HANDSHAKE METHOD

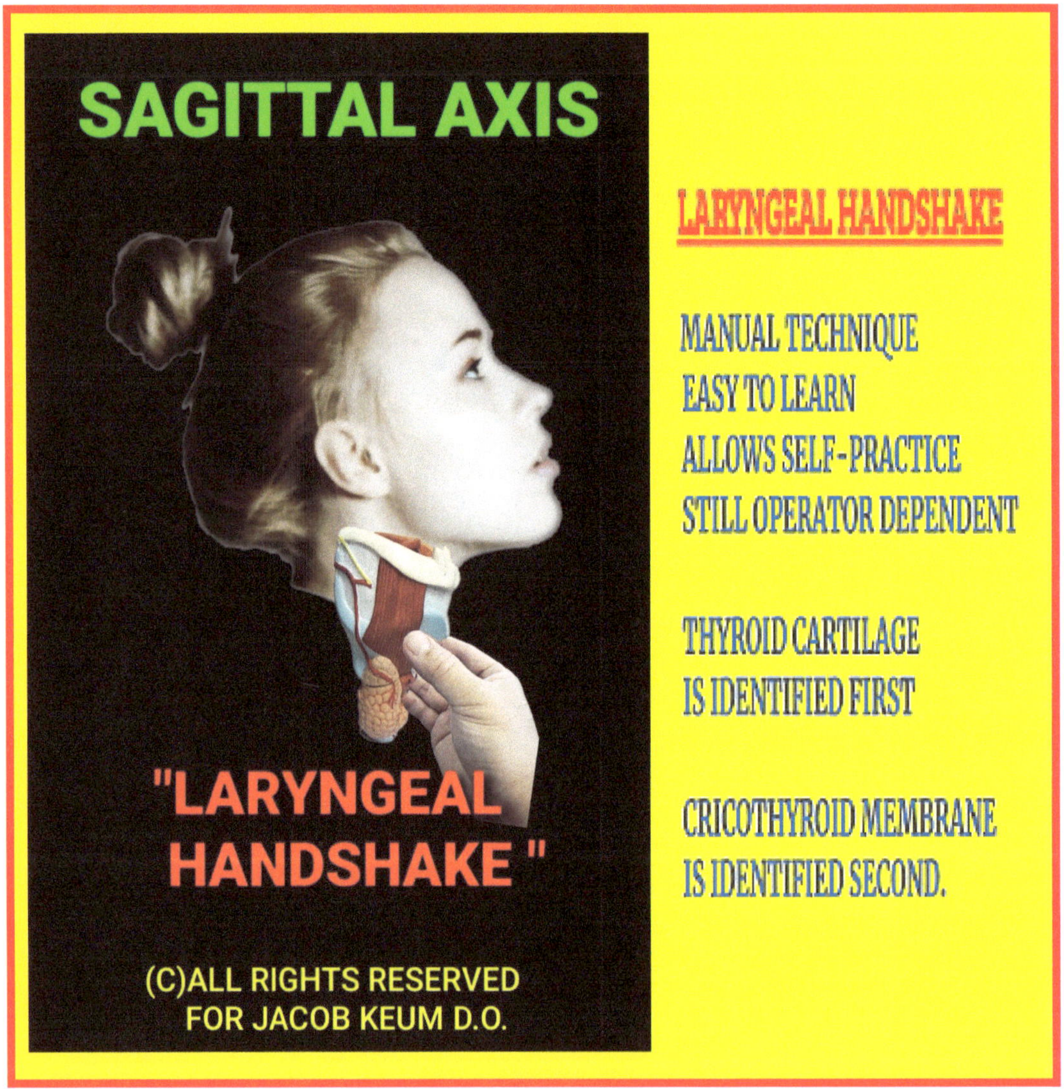

SAGITTAL AXIS

"LARYNGEAL HANDSHAKE "

(C)ALL RIGHTS RESERVED
FOR JACOB KEUM D.O.

LARYNGEAL HANDSHAKE

MANUAL TECHNIQUE
EASY TO LEARN
ALLOWS SELF-PRACTICE
STILL OPERATOR DEPENDENT

THYROID CARTILAGE
IS IDENTIFIED FIRST

CRICOTHYROID MEMBRANE
IS IDENTIFIED SECOND.

The Four Finger Width Technique

First, we use the dominant hand with four fingers closed linearly from index to 5th digit in 90 degree orientation. Second, we contact the suprasternal notch with the tip of 5th digit in 30 to 45° in the sagittal axis.

Third, while maintaining distal tip of 5th digit in contact with the suprasternal notch then tilt the hand directly forwards along the sagittal axis about 20 to 30°, then the tip of the index finger will contact the estimated location of the cricothyroid membrane. (21)

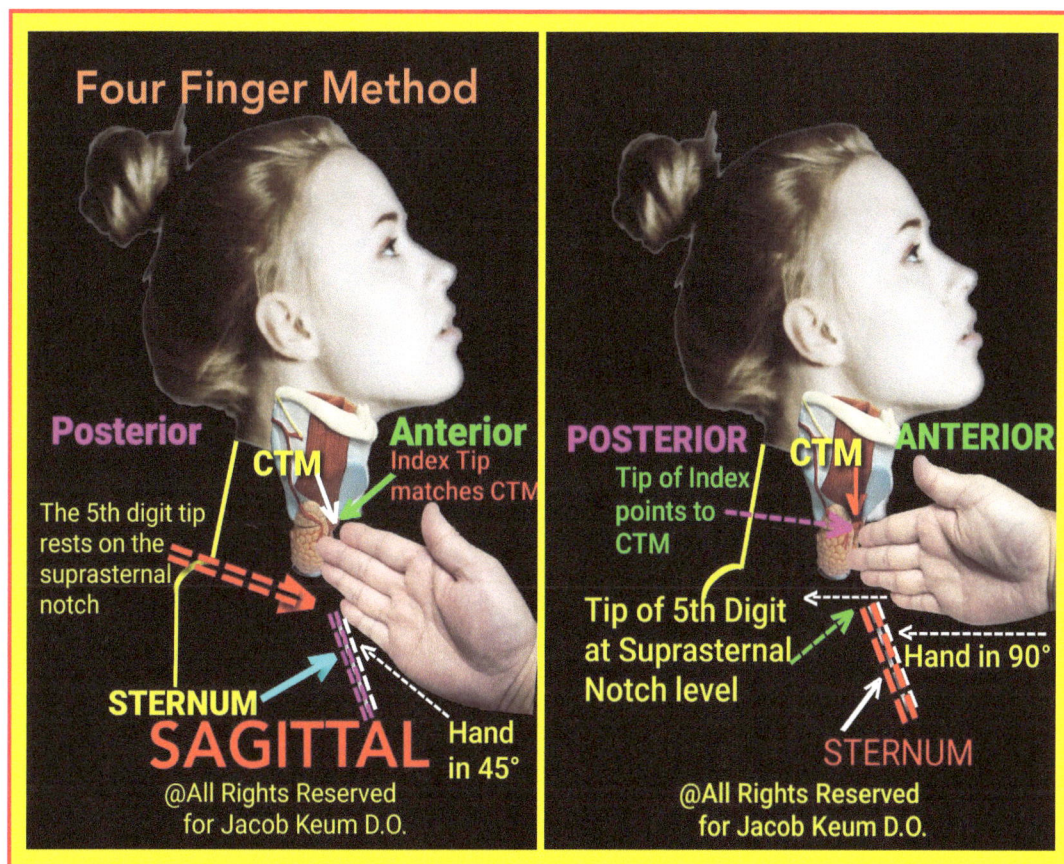

Please note: the Four Finger Width Method can lead to errors in accurately estimating the correct location of the Cricothyroid membrane since It does not take into account the variability in hand size of the operating surgeon versus the anatomical variability for individual patients with measurement differing in their neck sizes, age, gender, body frame, race, prior surgical scars and deformities. Also, there could be pre-existing airway deviations from tumors in the neck region that can lead to errors in anatomical landmark estimation leading to inaccurate localization of the cricothyroid membrane with significant complications from these errors during emergency airway surgical procedures. (21)(28)(44)(58)

There is a high degree of error when trying to confirm the accurate anatomical location of cricothyroid membrane when only the manual palpation is used under high time pressure. (12)(21)(33)(49)

FOUR FINGER WIDTH METHOD

ADVANTAGES

QUICK ESTIMATION
NO ULTRASOUND REQUIRED
EASY TO LEARN

DISADVANTAGES

POSSIBLY INACCURATE
NECK ANATOMY VARIANTS
SURGEON'S HAND SIZE VARIES

FOUR FINGER WIDTH METHOD

FOUR FINGER WIDTH METHOD STEPS:

1) With Dominant with 4 fingers closed, rest the tip of pinky finger on the suprasternal notch. (hand positioned along the sagittal plane)

2) Then, rotate the hand following The sagittal plane till the tip of index finger touches the anterior neck region.

3) The point of contact by the index finger tip will indicate the estimated location of the cricothyroid membrane

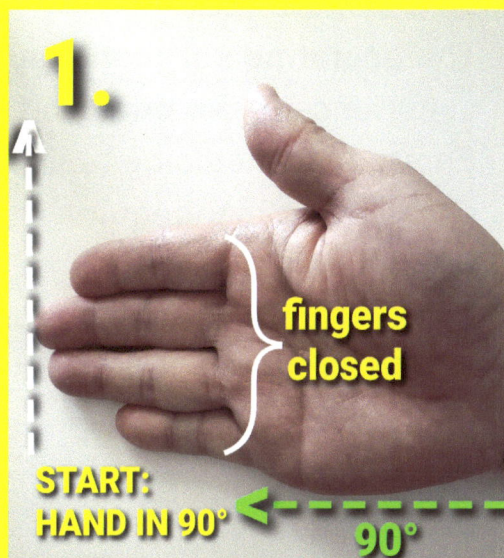

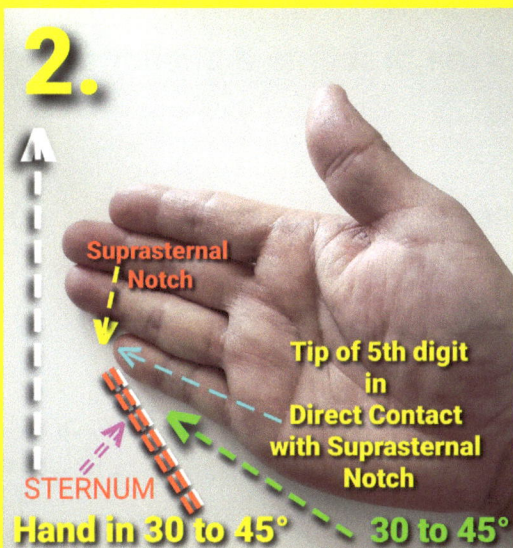

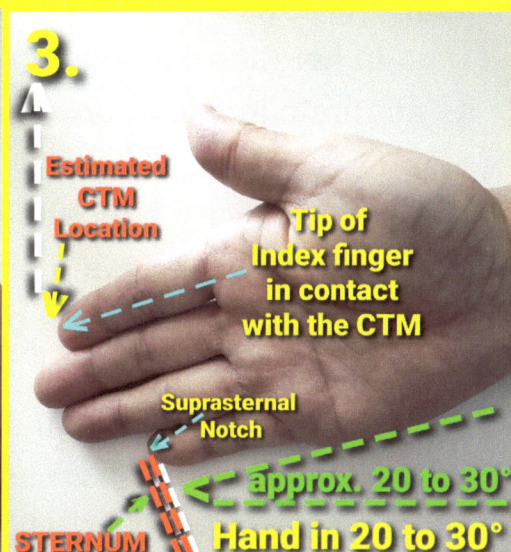

1.

fingers closed

START: HAND IN 90°

90°

2.

Suprasternal Notch

Tip of 5th digit in Direct Contact with Suprasternal Notch

STERNUM

Hand in 30 to 45°   30 to 45°

3.

Estimated CTM Location

Tip of Index finger in contact with the CTM

Suprasternal Notch

STERNUM

approx. 20 to 30°

Hand in 20 to 30°

CHALLENGING FACTORS OF THE CRICOTHYROIDOTOMY:

1. The procedure is performed under high stress and time restraints.

2. The operating surgeon may have little or complete lack of experience in the prior performance of cricothyroidotomy. Emergency Medicine residencies only require practice on cadavers or mannequins as part of completing their training requirements.
   The optimal competency for the procedure may be lacking due to the infrequent cases of airway obstruction requiring cricothyroidotomy.

3. Lack of familiarity with the anatomy of the cricothyroid membrane, and its small dimensions of approximately 1 cm in height and 0.8 cm in wide presents a challenge in its accurate localization. (42)(61)

4. The anatomy varies by gender, by race, by the neck adipose tissue density in obese patients, or with scars from prior surgeries or the presence of tumors altering the anatomy.(28)(37)(58)
   The accuracy of the manual palpatory findings leads only to approximately ⅓ of successful cricothyroidotomy without ultrasound guidance. (8)(12)(26)(28)(33)(57) And the ultrasound guidance localization is proven to improve the localization of the cricothyroid membrane. (29)

The ultrasound, unlike static imaging modalities such as MRI or CT, is also very capable of imaging dynamically important laryngeal structures which must be taken into consideration to prevent complications such as Injury to vocal cords and proximal vascular structures. (59)(60)

The following are images from the case report published by Okano, et al. highlighting the challenges of locating the cricothyroid membrane when the normal anatomy of the neck region is altered due to the presence of a tumor. In this case, the manual palpation led to errors in localization since the precise location of the cricothyroid membrane was deviated from the center axis or midline laterally.
The ultrasound guided localization was essential in performing the cricothyroidotomy in the correct location. (All images were published with permission from Doctors Kohji Uzawa, Joho Tokumine, and Okano's team at Kyorin University School of Medicine Tokyo, Japan.)

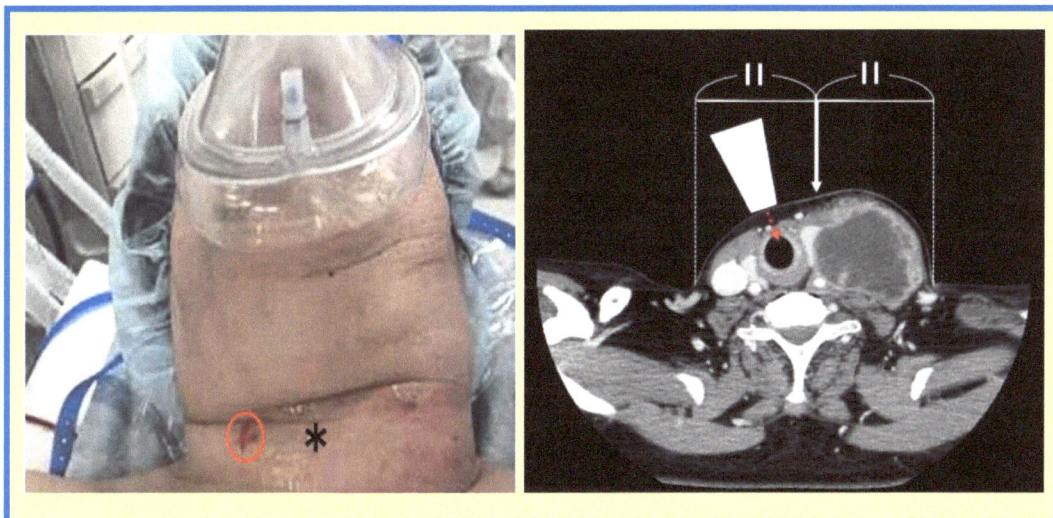

Left, a large neck tumor is seen. The CT scan shows the tumor.

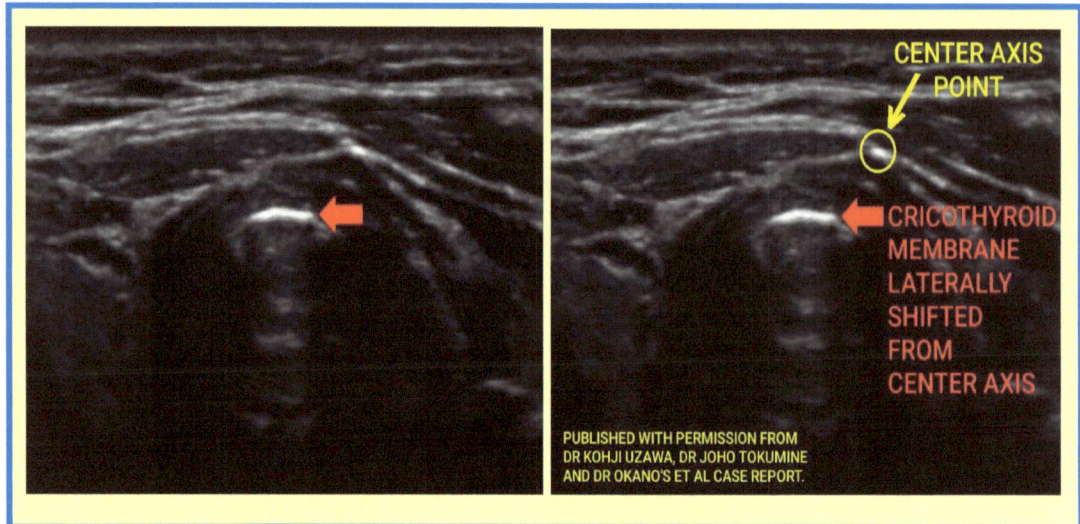

CENTER AXIS POINT

CRICOTHYROID MEMBRANE LATERALLY SHIFTED FROM CENTER AXIS

PUBLISHED WITH PERMISSION FROM DR KOHJI UZAWA, DR JOHO TOKUMINE AND DR OKANO'S ET AL CASE REPORT.

The red arrow shows the displaced cricothyroid membrane from the midline.

5. The lack of a simple systematic method to localize the cricothyroid membrane can lead to critical errors in anatomical position when only manual palpation is used leading to very significant complications during cricothyroidotomy. Surgical airway courses in residency programs dismiss the need to master the anatomical knowledge needed; even though we are very certain that 99% of this procedure is the actual correct localization of the cricothyroid membrane.(34)
    The ultrasound guided localization for trainees with only minimal experience with ultrasound could take longer to cannulate the cricothyroid membrane by more than 60 seconds but there is an increase in accuracy. (15)(49)(52) We believe there could be numerous factors for this time delay with ultrasound guided localization: Diagnostic Ultrasound machines take time to boot up to be ready for

scanning and the current difficult airway set up in most institutions do not include ultrasound readiness as part of their airway instruments tray setup. Also, the delayed decision in determining the necessity to use the ultrasound during difficult airway requiring surgical airway management and lack of proper familiarity with the scanning of cricothyroid membrane directly related to the lack of a proper scanning method or system. Very few trainees or even practicing airway surgeons are familiarized with localization systems, including the T-A-C-A technique. We are very optimistic that the scanning time specifically be reduced to 5 to 10 seconds with proper training and practice.

Even though our main goal in this book is the localization of cricothyroid membrane, we should at least discuss very briefly when and why the cricothyroidotomy would be required. Because the main objective of the ultrasound localization of cricothyroid membrane is to perform the cricothyroidotomy most expeditiously with minimal complications.

So here we will review the indications of the cricothyroidotomy. Some ultrasonographic images do cover some trachea on a limited basis in case tracheotomy is chosen instead of cricothyroidotomy.

The Indications for Surgical, Percutaneous, and Needle Cricothyroidotomy:

Facial trauma

Neck trauma

Anatomical variant (tumors, scars)(27)(28)(37)

Burn Injury

Anaphylaxis/Severe Angioedema

*Needle approach is reserved for

Pediatric Patients (younger than 11 years old) (27)

**All unable to intubate scenarios where patient is at risk of impending cardiopulmonary arrest.

The anatomical studies of cricothyroid membrane apply to adult patients and it can include pediatric patients from age 11 and older.

Those pediatric patients younger than 11 years old require a different anatomical references because of their much smaller size and manual palpatory localization. (53)

Even, in the pediatric emergency practice, the ultrasound guided localization of the cricothyroid membrane improves the accuracy of its identification with higher probability than the simple manual palpation methods. (35) (53)

Also, in the pediatric patients of these age group, surgical approaches using incision is not recommended due to complications in their development of these anatomical structures and the airway scarring as later complications in their lives.

In younger pediatric patients, high pressure oxygen delivery is achieved via percutaneous Needle device can be used as a rescue before definitive management is recommended. So they will get percutaneously inserted needle cricothyroidotomy as their main choice of management until the patient can be safely transferred to a regional pediatric hospital or tertiary center with availability of expert airway team capable of safely performing definitive airway, including tracheotomy. (30)

One caveat to this is high pressure oxygen delivery via needle is inspiratory in nature since it won't allow expiration process to occur so it is not a truly ventilatory system. CO_2 retention will occur because only oxygen is delivered via the needle and there is no way to allow CO_2 removal. As a result, the estimate is the high pressure oxygen delivery via needle inserted into the cricothyroid membrane is only a temporary bridge or rescue oxygenation-only system, not truly ventilatory. (27) By definition, the truly ventilatory system must achieve the inspiration and the expiration processes.

Typical Clinical Scenario For the Cricothyroidotomy:

"Can't intubate and can't ventilate"

In the ambulance call to the Emergency Department, the paramedics report that they are bringing a patient in acute respiratory distress with very poor oxygen saturation. They also report they were not able to intubate due to possible obstruction during their intubation attempt. (64)

The paramedics are also reporting they are having difficulty manually ventilating this patient due to resistance in manual bagging or ventilation via ball valve mask device.

As the Emergency Medicine provider on the receiving end, based on paramedics report you determine that this a typical scenario of "Can't intubate, can't ventilate."
The following critical thinking should come to your mind:

1) There is a high probability of <u>airway obstruction</u>.

2) There must be complex emergency airway management preparation protocols in place which must include:
   a. Crash cart containing standard intubation equipment.
   b. Surgical airway cart with the ultrasound to be ready to scan the neck. Ultrasound devices require booting time to be ready for immediate use. Frequent protocols must be in place to make sure the ultrasound machine is fully charged and ready to go at all times when needed.

During these steps, an attempt should be made to intubate regardless if the obstruction was or was not verified by paramedics or other providers. There is always a chance that in a new attempt by a different provider the successful intubation can be completed.

Now, if the upper airway obstruction is also observed in the new intubation attempt then we can quickly proceed to surgical, percutaneous or needle cricothyroidotomy without delay, since cardiac arrest from respiratory arrest can occur very rapidly. (64)
It is wise to have a surgical airway tray ready for immediate access to surgical instrumentation for use and, in our method, having the diagnostic ultrasound ready for scan will aid in reducing the overall procedure time. We advocate that the ultrasound be turned on and ready for immediate scanning for cricothyroid membrane localization towards the execution of cricothyroidotomy without delay. The reliability of the scanning equipment is an essential part of the preparation.

We prefer the ultrasound scanning probe be directly connected via hardwire than the wireless connection. Unfortunately, while a wireless probe can add convenience, it lacks the connection reliability, especially in critical clinical applications.

And with the complex airway set up in place, we can scan immediately with ultrasound to locate the cricothyroid membrane first in the most expeditious manner. With practice, we can locate the cricothyroid membrane with ultrasound in 5 seconds using the most rapid scanning technique called the 2 axis verification 1-2-1 system. In the preparation of this book, I reviewed the published works on localization by Vanderbilt ER, UMDNJ ER and T-A-C-A technique. I will not review all these methods at this time, but I would like to discuss Kristensen's T-A-C-A technique in order to highlight some differences in the methodology. (9)

Among all the proponents of localization of the cricothyroid membrane, Kristensen et al. published a very comprehensive review and they created the T-A-C-A technique. (9) Its acronym is easy to remember but it does not provide the visual confirmation in different axis views in its technique. The T-A-C-A technique in all its steps emphasizes the transverse axis view only. (9) Later, Kristensen et al. did publish the scanning time differences for the transverse axis and sagittal or longitudinal axis scans, but it did not modify the T-A-C-A technique to incorporate the sagittal axis confirmation. (51)

The airway surgeons will have to initiate the first incision without being able to visualize the important anatomical landmarks in the sagittal axis. So, the simple and most easy way to remember would be a scanning sequence that follows this traditional palpatory sequence with confirmatory step in the different axis view such as the sagittal axis of the cricothyroid membrane.

As a radiology principle, the ability to visualize the same structure from different axis views can add very valuable information about the anatomical landmark of interest. For example, you will see that one view X-rays yield limited information based on only one dimension while two-view or even three-view x-rays add a rather more complete picture with more dimensional information. This could even disclose an injury which would otherwise go undetected in the one view. I suspect that scanning speed can be a significant constraint; but with extensive practice, the localization scanning can be reduced to 5 to 10 seconds of total scanning time.

Once experienced, the practitioner will be able to locate and confirm the cricothyroid membrane location with two views only.

Now, we are going to explain the The T-A-C-A technique which aims to identify the structures with ultrasound in following sequence:

1. **Thyroid cartilage**
2. **Cricothyroid membrane seen with airline**
3. **Cricoid scan**
4. **Cricothyroid membrane (returning to step 2)**

The T-A-C-A scanning technique is intended as the most expedited emergency scanning technique for the practitioner who had sufficient practice and familiarity in ultrasound scanning of the neck region.

One important weakness of the T-A-C-A ultrasound technique is the lack of additional confirmatory in sagittal view.
It is a 4 step localization technique with possible loss of time.

As I have stated before that ultimately the scanning system should allow the airway surgeon to be able to confirm the precise location of the Cricothyroid Membrane with 2 scanning views in about 5 to 10 seconds.

The best way to achieve this mastery is to first practice a more comprehensive scanning protocol, including the TSTS and 5S scanning methodologies. They will help all providers to get familiarized with key ultrasonographic anatomical landmarks first and foremost.

It can also help in the process to become very well-trained in correctly identify the important neck airway anatomy with palpation as well since you have the ability to confirm your tactile findings with the ultrasound scanning.

We are going to present 5 scanning protocols and

The Paperclip Shadow Confirmation Method:
(Easy mnemonics with new ultrasound correlations)

1. **TSTS Scanning Protocol**
2. **5S Scanning Protocol**
3. **Quick 2 axis Confirmation Protocol**
4. **Quick 2 Axis with Procedure View Protocol (1-2-1)**
5. **TC-CTM 2xP Scanning Protocol**

***Paperclip Shadow Confirmation Method (a review)**

It is expected that once you become very familiarized with the precise identification of all anatomical structures of interest, your palpatory and ultrasound localizing skills of the cricothyroid membrane will improve, giving you, the airway surgeon, the option to do the cricothyroidotomy with greater confidence. This can be achieved either by manual palpation technique or ultrasound-guided technique or the combination of both, if he or she chooses to do so.

Chapter 2

Equipment

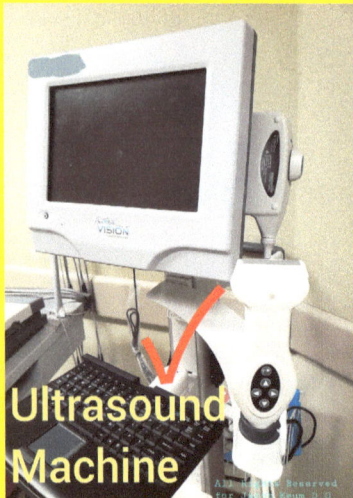

A. Basic Diagnostic Ultrasound Machine.
(Site Rite Vision by Bard)

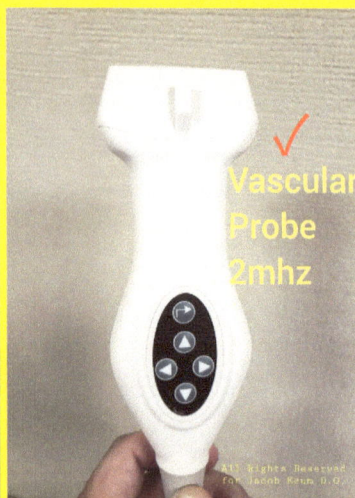

B1. Vascular Probe 2 MHz (flat surface)

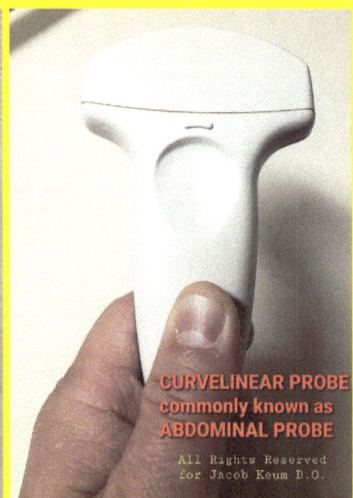

B2. Abdominal or Curvilinear Probe*
(*instead of vascular probe)

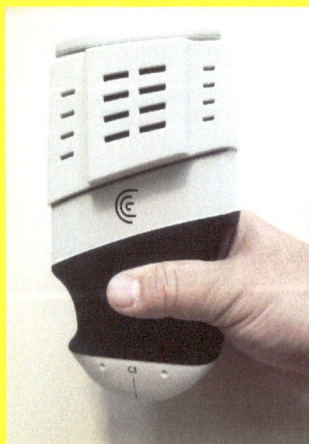

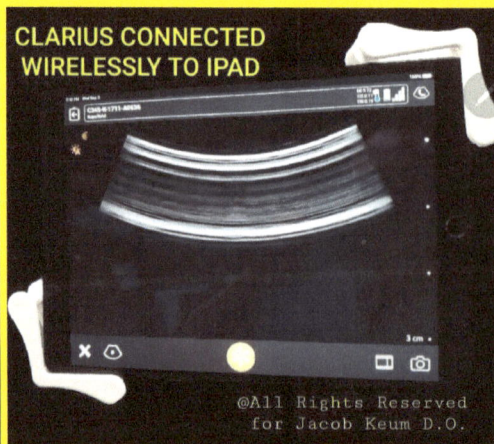

A.C3HD Probe. (By Clarius, Canada) **B. WIRELESSLY CONNECTED IPAD.** (Ipad tablet by Apple San Jose, California) **C.Scanning Gel**

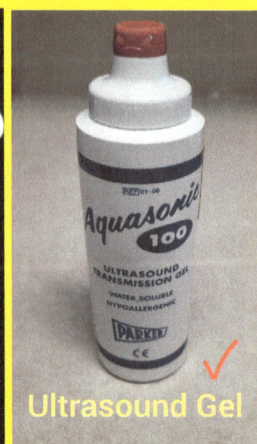

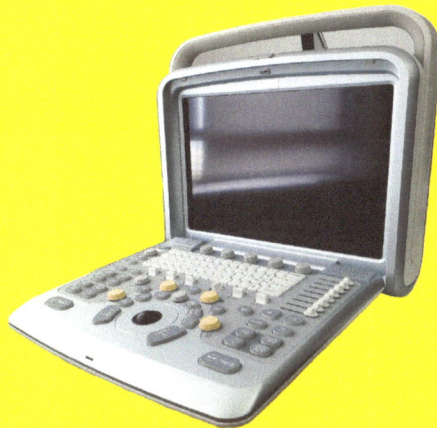

A. CHISON Q9 4D System.
   (CHISON by China)

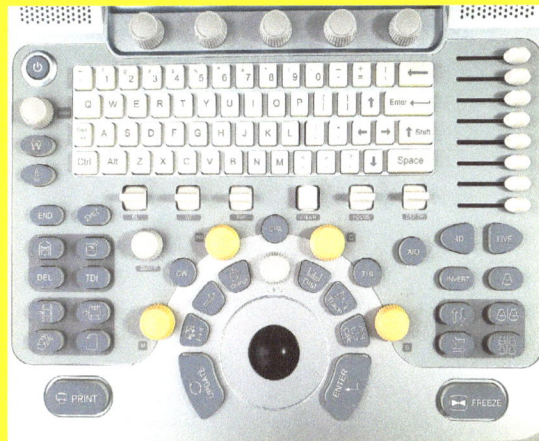

B. CHISON Q9 Control Panel

All functional, reliable diagnostic ultrasound machines with acceptable resolution can be used to do this scanning. We prefer hard-wired probes over wirelessly connected one due to critical usage of these devices. The vascular probe or linear probe is the preferred probe to scan these structures, however when the vascular probe is not available then the curvilinear probe (abdominal) can also be used to scan the CRICOTHYROID MEMBRANE. (with the curvilinear probe, the CRICOTHYROID MEMBRANE will look as CURVED shape). With the vascular probe, the cricothyroid membrane is seen as STRAIGHT or LINEARLY shaped.

VASCULAR PROBE
(LINEAR OR STRAIGHT)

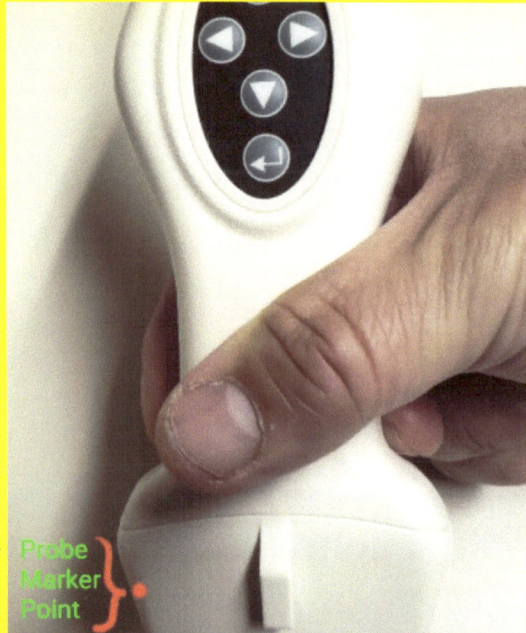

VASCULAR PROBE

CEPHALAD
<===

CAUDAL
===>
CRICOID

Superior Border

Inferior Border

THYROID CARTILAGE

Cricothyroid Membrane looks STRAIGHT

SAGITTAL

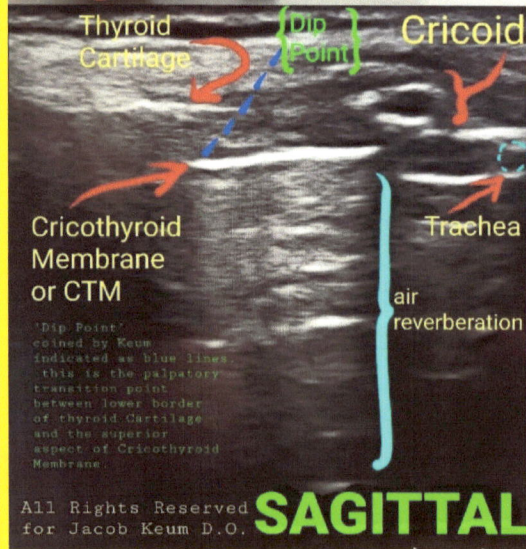

Thyroid Cartilage

{Dip Point}

Cricoid

Cricothyroid Membrane or CTM

Trachea

air reverberation

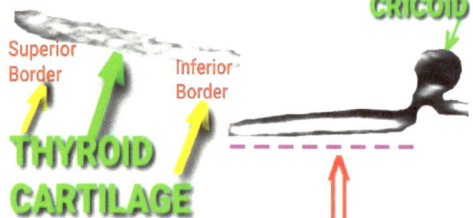

'Dip Point' coined by Keum indicated as blue lines this is the palpatory transition point between lower border of thyroid Cartilage and the superior aspect of Cricothyroid Membrane.

SAGITTAL

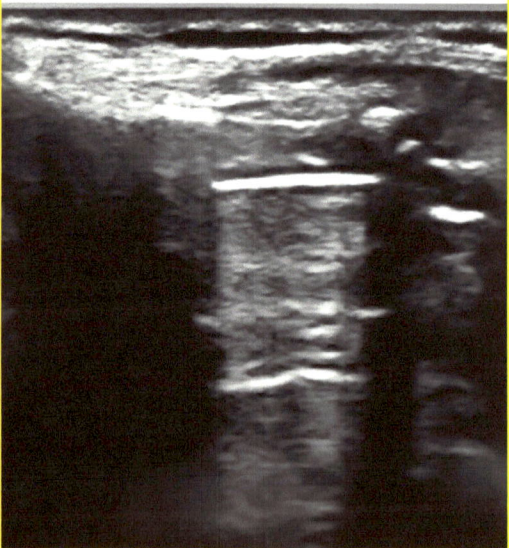

The vascular or linear probe will yield a more linear or straight view of the imaged structures.

ABDOMINAL PROBE (CURVILINEAR)

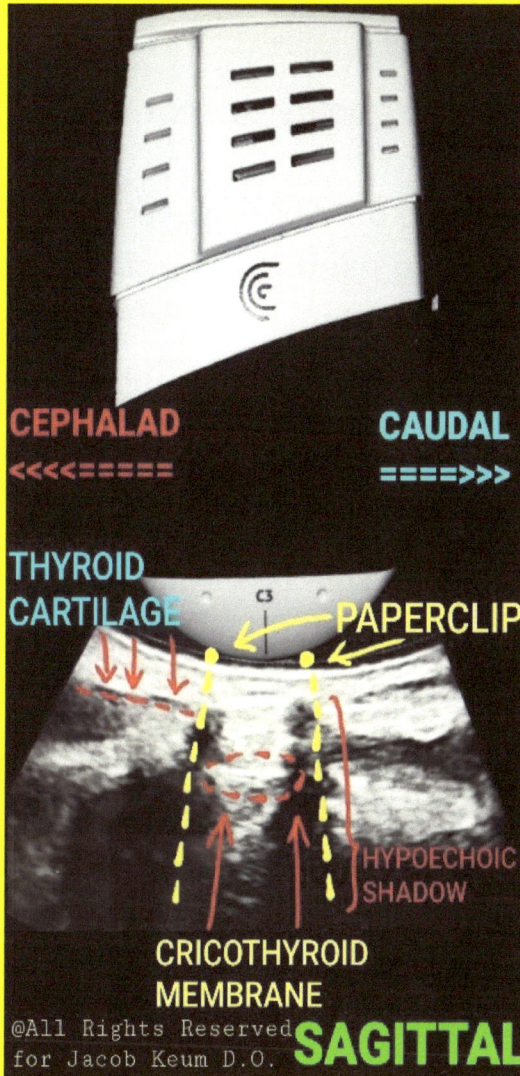

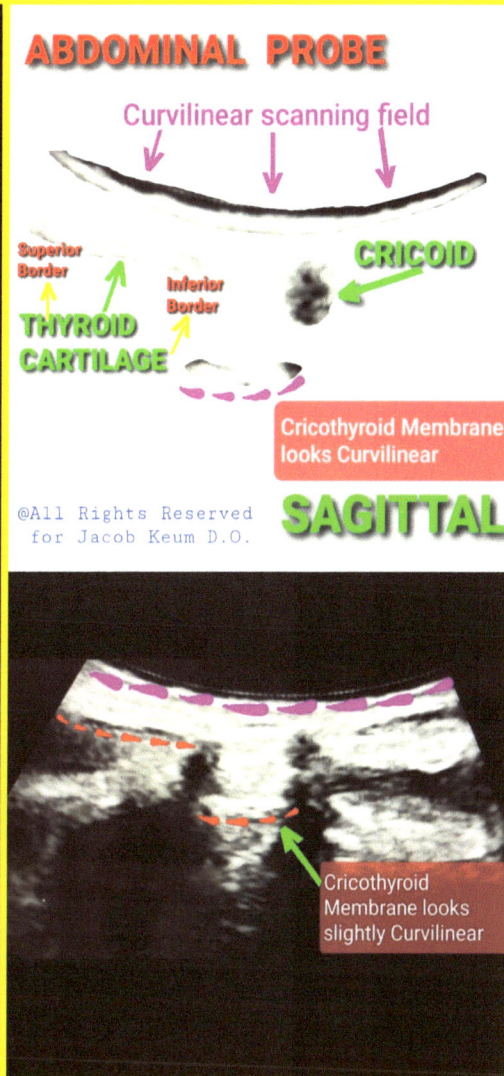

CEPHALAD
<<<<======

CAUDAL
====>>>

THYROID CARTILAGE

PAPERCLIP

HYPOECHOIC SHADOW

CRICOTHYROID MEMBRANE

SAGITTAL

ABDOMINAL PROBE

Curvilinear scanning field

CRICOID

Superior Border

Inferior Border

THYROID CARTILAGE

Cricothyroid Membrane looks Curvilinear

SAGITTAL

Cricothyroid Membrane looks slightly Curvilinear

The multipurpose curvilinear probe is more commonly seen in abdominal probes and you can see that the same structures seen with the vascular probe before now these same structures appear more curvilinear in shape as well.

Ultrasound Scanning Settings

It is important to spend some time learning about the scanning settings of your ultrasound machine. When I refer to settings, we are talking about particular basic adjustments you can make in the machine to improve the overall quality of your images (image optimization).
We are not going to go into extensive details over settings since with most ultrasound machines being used in the point of care settings, the adjustments are already set in a way minimize changes in adjustments that are needed to obtain the quality scanned images.

I will briefly discuss the following adjustments to be done to obtain acceptable scanned images. This is a quick synopsis. It is not intended to replace the entire field of knobology.

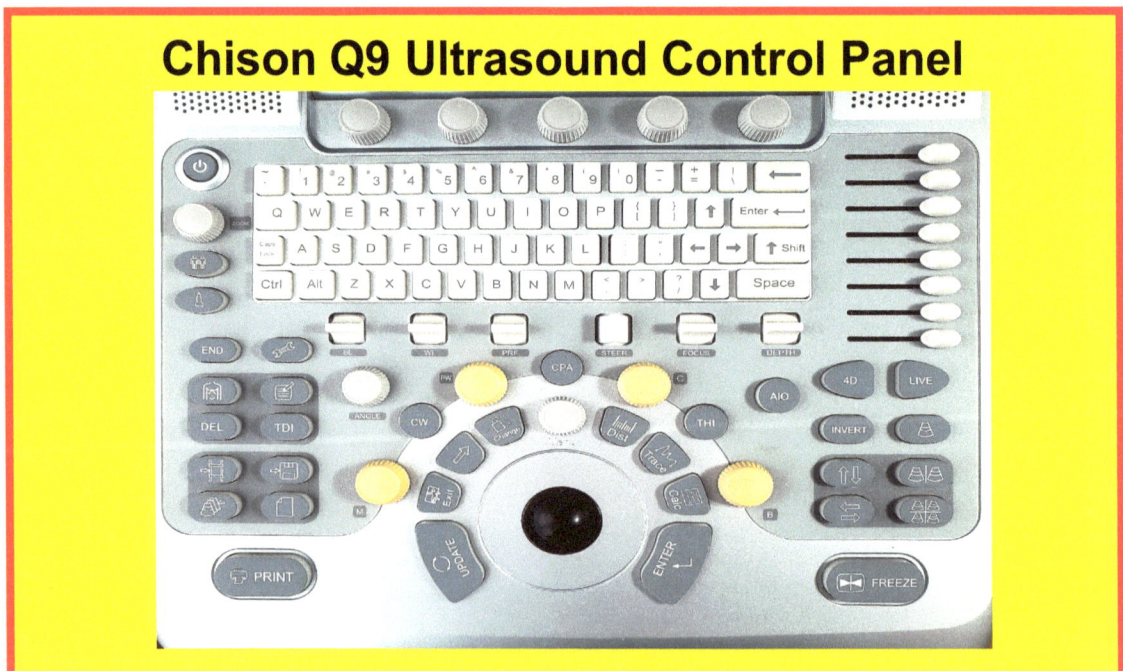

Chison Q9 Ultrasound Control Panel

Frequency:

Higher frequency gives higher resolution
But the depth of scanning field will be shallow
Lower frequency gives lower resolution
But the depth of scanning field will be deeper
The vascular probe is high frequency 2 to 3 mhz.(48)
The abdominal probe is 3.5 to 6 mhz.(22, 48)

Depth: Adjustable scanning depth in cm
Vascular probe (1 to 6cm)
Abdominal probe (6 to 10cm)

Gain: This is the process of signal amplification
Higher signal gain creates brighter images
Lower signal gain creates darker images. (24)

THE THREE EXAMPLES OF GAIN SETTINGS:

Too much gain(darker) Too little gain(brighter) Balanced gain

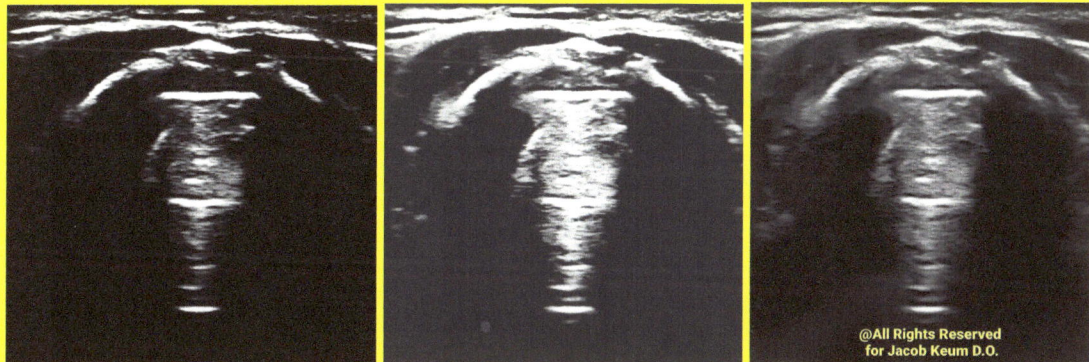

TGC or Time Gain Compensation

There are multiple control knobs used to adjust the gain at different depths so that the final image has uniform quality by increasing or decreasing the returning ultrasound signal strength to compensate for tissue attenuation and depth. (26)

TGC Controls

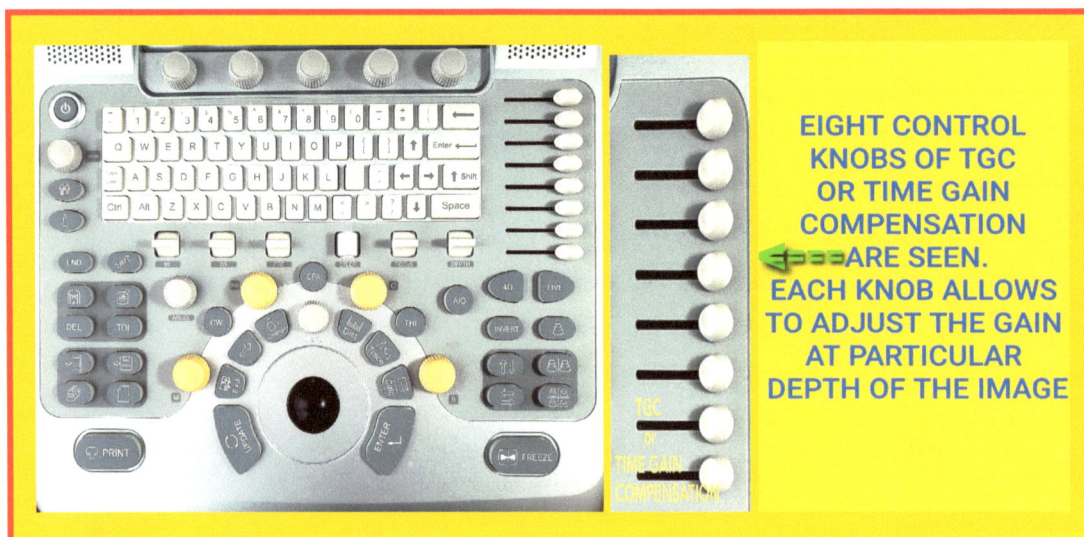

EIGHT CONTROL KNOBS OF TGC OR TIME GAIN COMPENSATION ARE SEEN. EACH KNOB ALLOWS TO ADJUST THE GAIN AT PARTICULAR DEPTH OF THE IMAGE

B Mode

is the scanned image display modality when images are created from 2 dimensions by using different scales of brightness of grey. (23)

We will only mention the B mode which will be the main mode to be used in our scanning sessions.

Color Flow Doppler

This feature in the settings can be very helpful, especially if you want to identify blood vessels and their locations near the structures of your interest. This particular feature paints with different colors to help identify what is a vein versus what is an artery. Its physical principle is based on the ultrasound beam signal reflections from the red blood cells flowing within the blood vessels. The velocity and direction of signal moving towards or away from the transducer or probe will determine the color that is displayed.

Blood flow away from the probe looks blue while blood flow towards the probe will look orange to red. (38)(40)

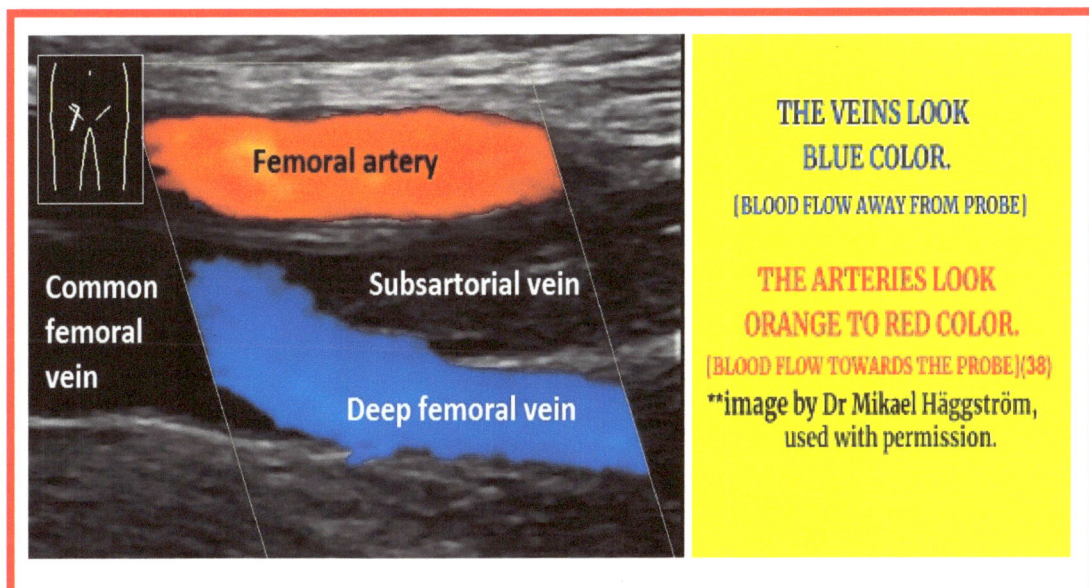

THE VEINS LOOK BLUE COLOR.
[BLOOD FLOW AWAY FROM PROBE]

THE ARTERIES LOOK ORANGE TO RED COLOR.
[BLOOD FLOW TOWARDS THE PROBE](38)
**image by Dr Mikael Häggström, used with permission.

Those wishing to pursue in depth study of the knobology or the subject dedicated to obtaining the best possible scanned ultrasound images should be making the best adjustments of the image with fine manipulation image variables with the multiple knobs and control setting levels. (25) (40) See references listed for further study.
You should spend enough time practicing the optimal settings during the scanning practice sessions to obtain the best image quality possible.

The best way to learn how to properly adjust the Image quality is spending extensive time with the ultrasound scanner settings in scanning sessions.

Chapter 3

Anatomical Landmarks Visuals

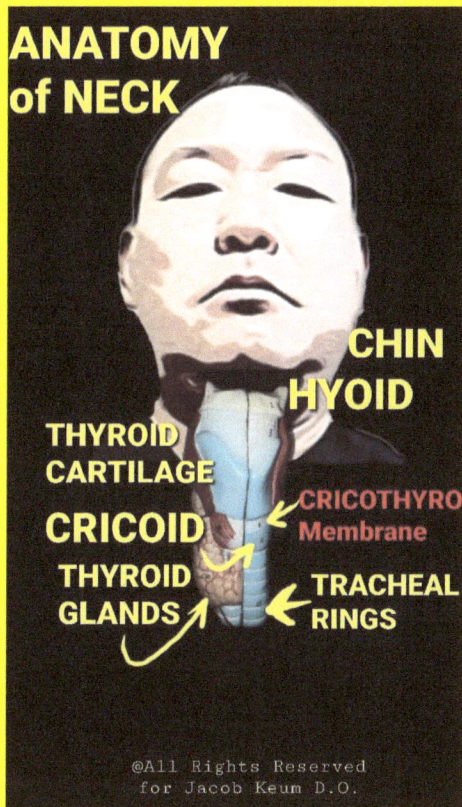

ANATOMY of NECK

CHIN
HYOID
THYROID CARTILAGE
CRICOID
THYROID GLANDS
CRICOTHYROID Membrane
TRACHEAL RINGS

@All Rights Reserved for Jacob Keum D.O.

SEQUENCE

1. CHIN
2. HYOID
3. THYROID CARTILAGE
4. CRICOTHYROID MEMBRANE
5. CRICOID
6. THYROID GLANDS
7. TRACHEAL RINGS

Identify all anatomical structures in sequence from the cephalad to caudal position (head to toe direction) using all modalities: visual, manual and ultrasound forms of structural identification from the chin to the most inferiorly located trachea.

1)CHIN=>2)HYOID=>3)THYROID CARTILAGE=> 4)CRICOTHYROID MEMBRANE=>5)CRICOID=> 6)TRACHEAL RINGS AND 7)THYROID GLANDS.

Front Center/Anterior View

ANATOMY
of NECK

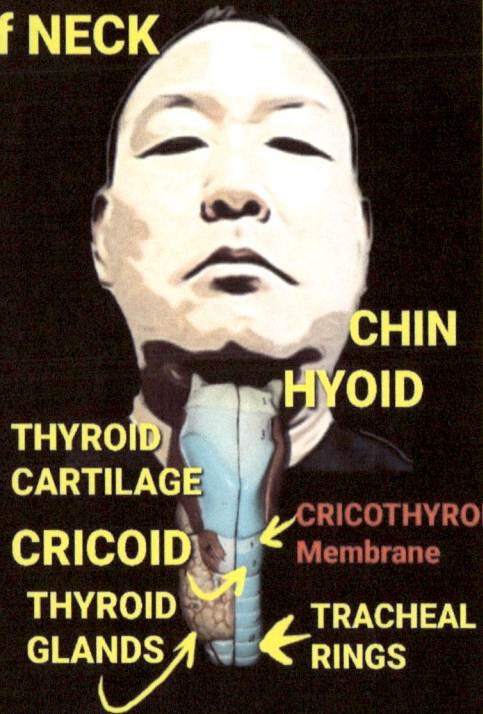

CHIN
HYOID

THYROID
CARTILAGE

CRICOID

CRICOTHYROID
Membrane

THYROID
GLANDS

TRACHEAL
RINGS

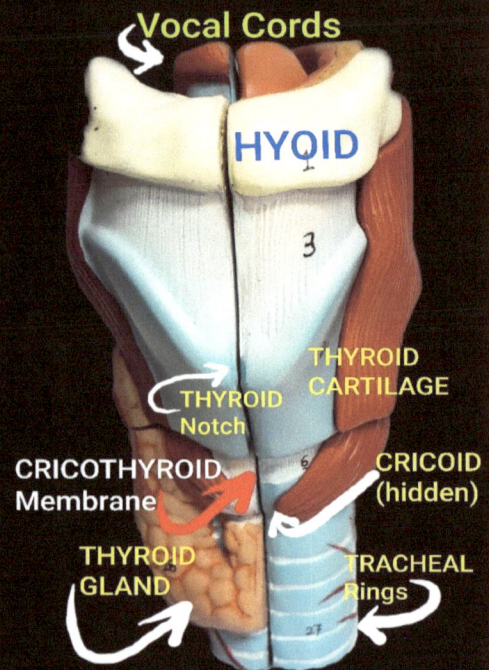

@All Rights Reserved
for Jacob Keum D.O.

ANTERIOR

Vocal Cords

HYOID

3

THYROID
Notch

THYROID
CARTILAGE

CRICOTHYROID
Membrane

CRICOID
(hidden)

THYROID
GLAND

TRACHEAL
Rings

@All Rights Reserved
for Jacob Keum D.O.

1) CHIN =>   2)HYOID =>
3) THYROID CARTILAGE =>
4) <u>CRICOTHYROID MEMBRANE</u> =>
5) CRICOID =>
6) THYROID GLANDS LATERALLY =>
7) TRACHEAL RINGS

Sagittal Axis/Lateral Left View

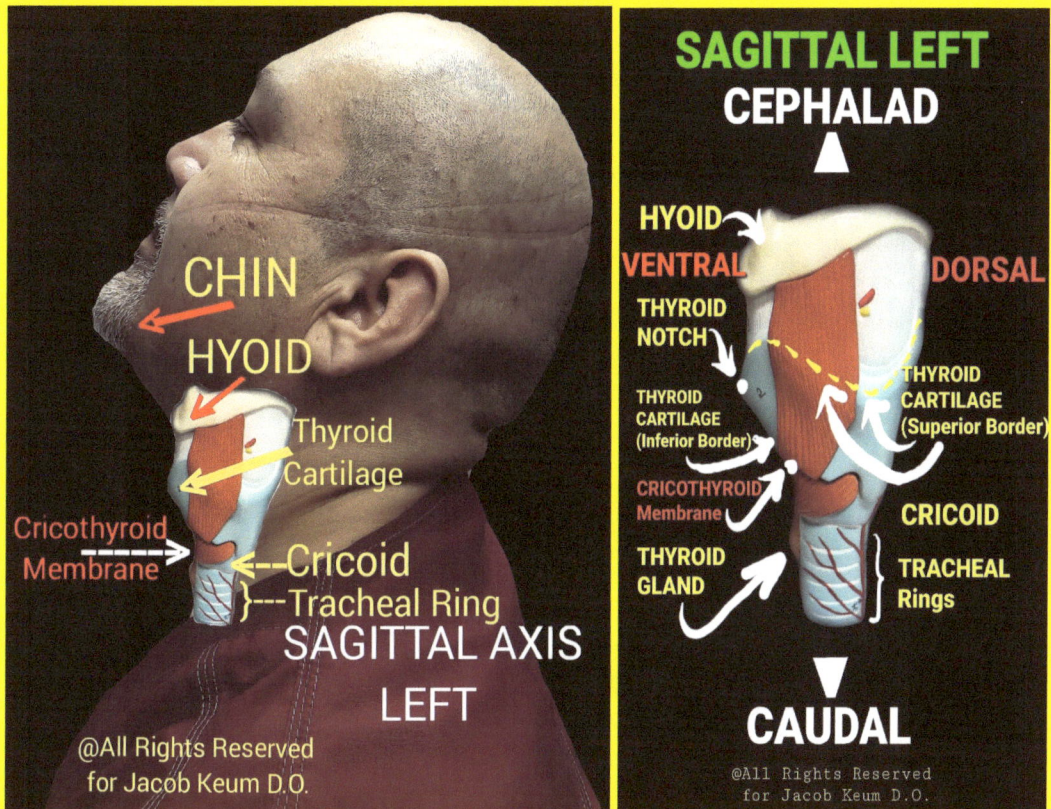

SAGITTAL LEFT

CEPHALAD

HYOID

VENTRAL — DORSAL

THYROID NOTCH

THYROID CARTILAGE (Inferior Border)

THYROID CARTILAGE (Superior Border)

CRICOTHYROID Membrane

CRICOID

THYROID GLAND

TRACHEAL Rings

CAUDAL

CHIN

HYOID

Thyroid Cartilage

Cricothyroid Membrane

Cricoid

Tracheal Ring

SAGITTAL AXIS LEFT

PALPATE THE CHIN FIRST
THEN CONTINUE WITH

=> HYOID (deeper plane slightly lower than Chin)

=> THYROID CARTILAGE

=> FALSE VOCAL CORD (Higher, not palpable)

=> TRUE VOCAL CORD (Lower, not palpable)

==>CRICOTHYROID MEMBRANE

==>CRICOID ===> TRACHEAL RINGS

Sagittal Axis/Lateral Right View

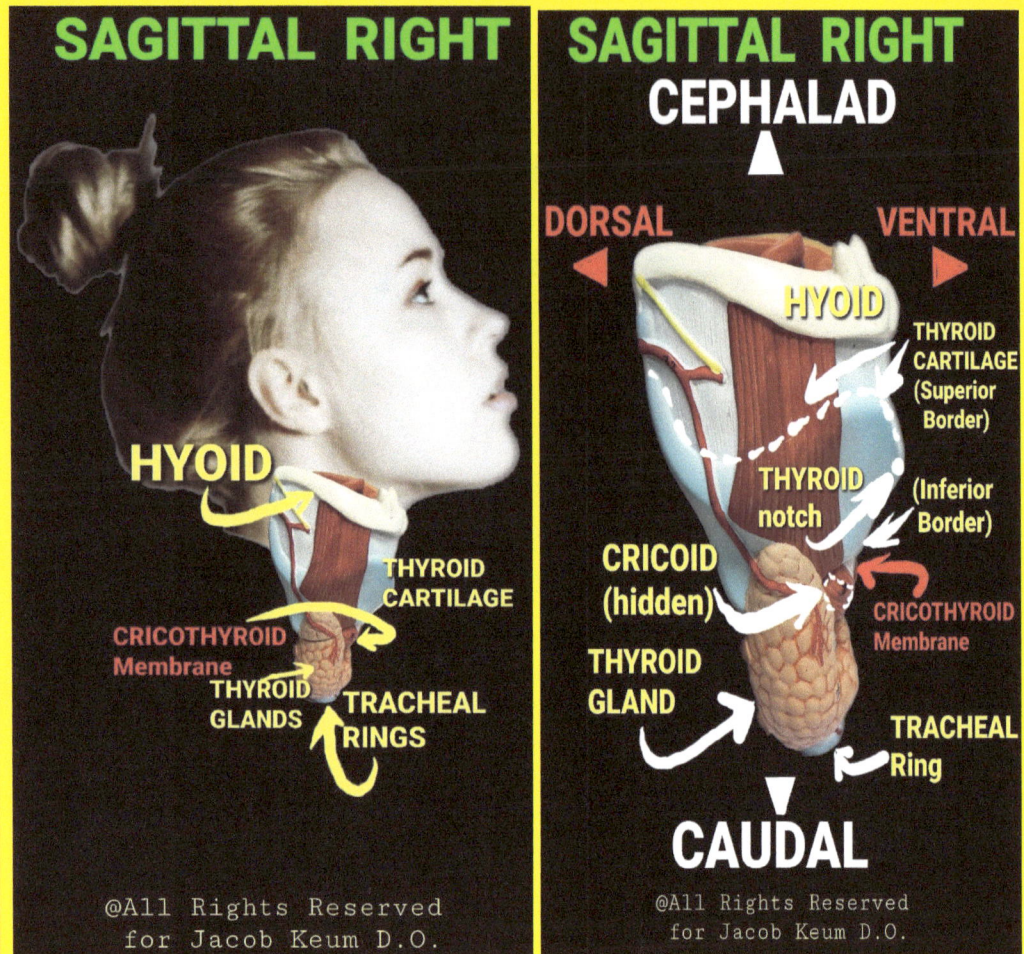

SAGITTAL RIGHT

HYOID

THYROID CARTILAGE

CRICOTHYROID Membrane

THYROID GLANDS

TRACHEAL RINGS

@All Rights Reserved for Jacob Keum D.O.

SAGITTAL RIGHT

CEPHALAD

DORSAL

VENTRAL

HYOID

THYROID CARTILAGE (Superior Border)

THYROID notch

(Inferior Border)

CRICOID (hidden)

THYROID GLAND

CRICOTHYROID Membrane

TRACHEAL Ring

CAUDAL

@All Rights Reserved for Jacob Keum D.O.

The manual palpation paired with ultrasound visualization add a very precise anatomical understanding.
Your first incision site in cricothyroidotomy will be more accurate. The ultrasound guidance transforms a basically blind procedure into a visual procedure with improved accuracy. (33)

Chapter 4

Ultrasound Anatomical Landmarks

First palpate the chin, then moving your fingers inferiorly in deeper and in slightly lower plane of palpation, you can find the hyoid bone which can be easily confused as the superior border of the thyroid cartilage. This error in palpation can risk injury to the vocal cord during the initial Incision for the surgical cricothyroidotomy. (42)

Some reported moderate difficulties in visualizing the hyoid with the ultrasound even when sublingual scanning modalities. (43) Contrary to reports, we are able to scan the hyoid with good resolution. The hyoid is seen as a bright signal with curvilinear shape in the scans.

**IT IS CRITICAL : DO NOT MISTAKE THE HYOID BONE With THYROID CARTILAGE TO AVOID VOCAL CORD INJURY.

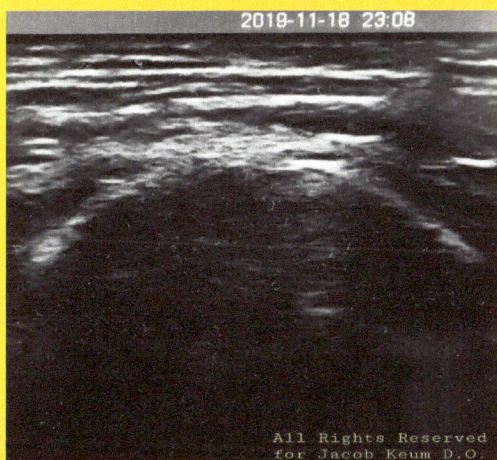

2018-11-18 23:08

HYOID

- SLIGHTLY INFERIOR TO CHIN
- FOUND IN DEEPER PLANE
- SUPERIOR TO THYROID CARTILAGE
- INVERTED SALAD BOWL LOOKING IN ULTRASOUND

HYOID ⇐ ("INVERTED SALAD BOWL")

HYOID SEEN AS
"INVERTED SALAD BOWL"

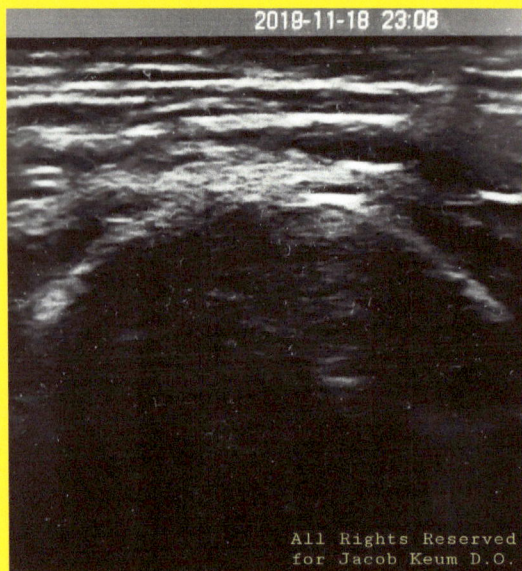

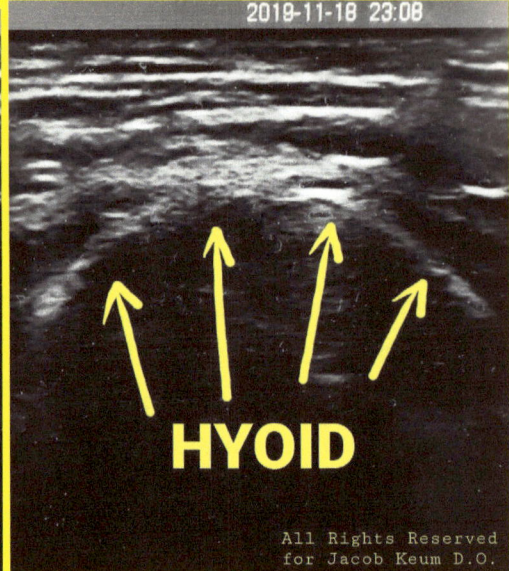

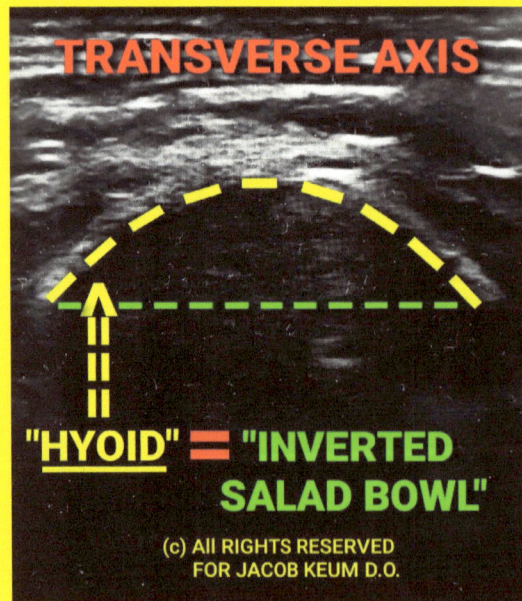

2018-11-18 23:08

2018-11-18 23:08

HYOID

TRANSVERSE AXIS

"HYOID" = "INVERTED SALAD BOWL"

HYOID

LOOKS LIKE
AN "INVERTED SALAD BOWL".

WHEN AN IMAGINARY LINE
IS CONNECTED IN THE ENDS
OF THE HYOID IN ULTRASOUND

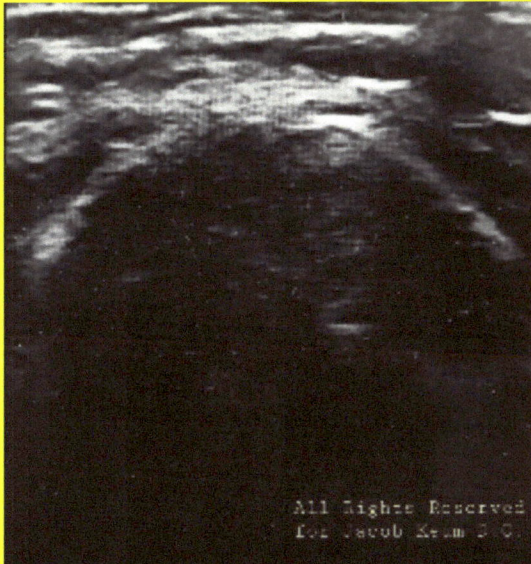

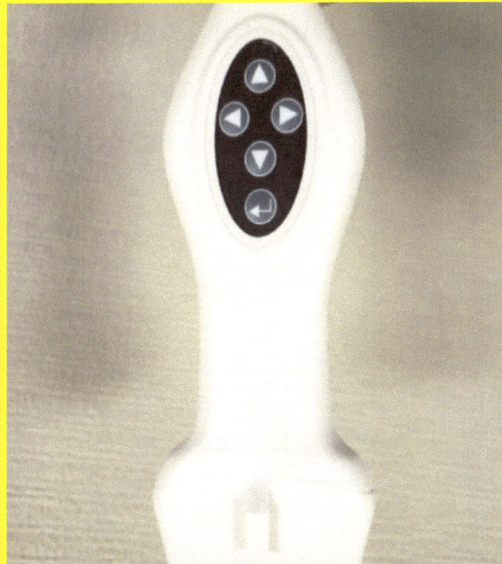

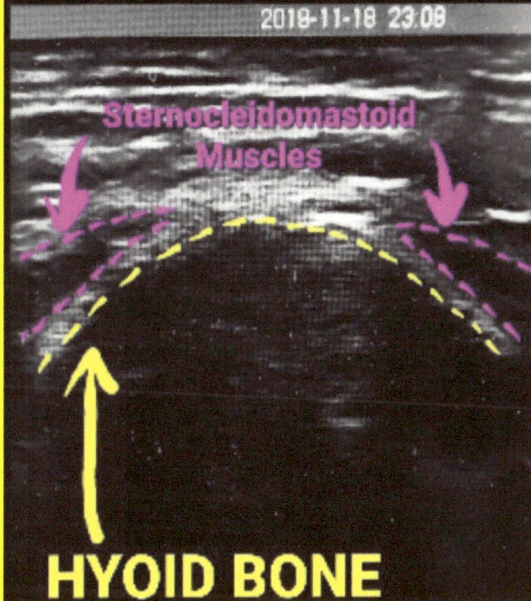

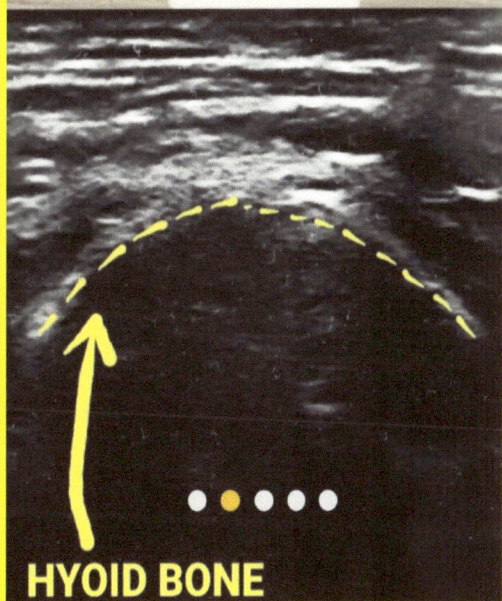

a.TRANSVERSE

b. WITH PROBE

THYROID CARTILAGE
(ALSO KNOWN AS "INVERTED V SHAPE")

The thyroid cartilage is located inferior to the hyoid. With the superior border of the thyroid cartilage at its front center, you will find what has been known as "Adam's Apple" which refers to the thyroid notch.

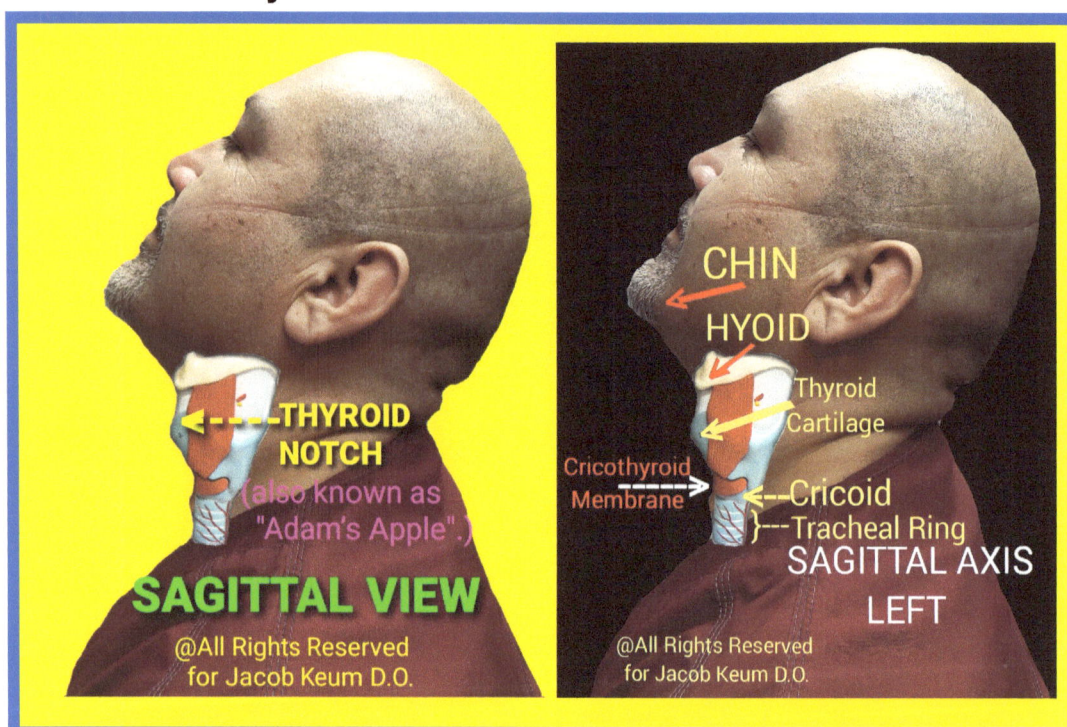

The thyroid notch, also known as the Adam's Apple, is more prominent in males. This anatomical location is the manual palpatory reference point that most operating surgeons attempt to manually palpate first in the process of identifying the SUPERIOR PART OF THYROID CARTILAGE in order to slide the fingers down along the anterior walls of the thyroid cartilage in order to locate the cricothyroid membrane, in order to perform the cricothyroidotomy.

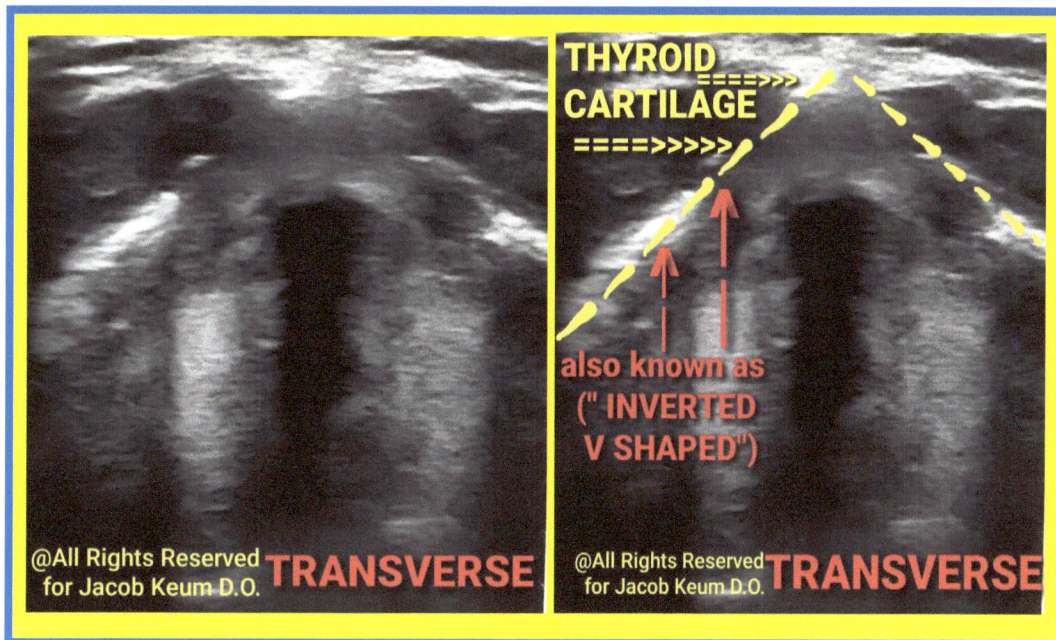

THYROID CARTILAGE
SEEN AS
"INVERTED V SHAPED"

Once, you see the INVERTED V SHAPED in the scan, you can identify this structure: the SUPERIOR BORDER OF THYROID CARTILAGE.

This is a key anatomical landmark in the localization process of the cricothyroid membrane.

1. Once you visually identify the INVERTED V SHAPED you know with greater certainty that you are looking at the SUPERIOR BORDER OF THE THYROID CARTILAGE.

Also by visually recognizing the SUPERIOR BORDER OF THE THYROID CARTILAGE you can be highly certain that you are below the plane where the hyoid bone is located.

2. Now you know that the hyoid is located above the "INVERTED V SHAPE" or SUPERIOR BORDER OF THE THYROID CARTILAGE.

3. Also, by correctly identifying with the ultrasound the "INVERTED V SHAPE" as the SUPERIOR BORDER OF THYROID CARTILAGE, you will also know the exact location of the false and true vocal cords.

By knowing this precise anatomical relationship, you can prevent a very critical cricothyroidotomy-associated complication which is mistaking the hyoid with the thyroid cartilage and making the incorrect Incision point between the hyoid and above the superior aspect of thyroid cartilage, which can injure the vocal cords.

THYROID CARTILAGE
AND PERTINENT STRUCTURES:

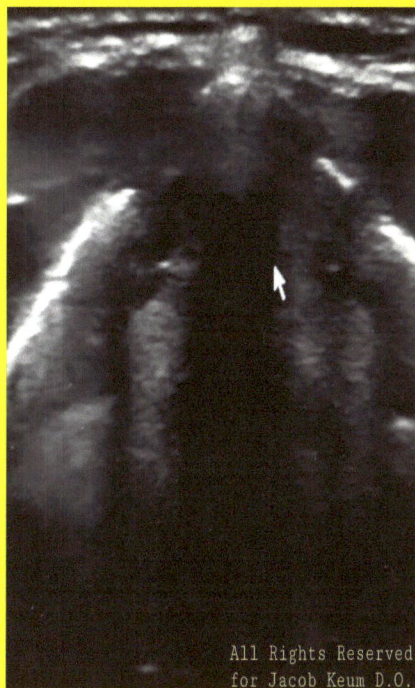

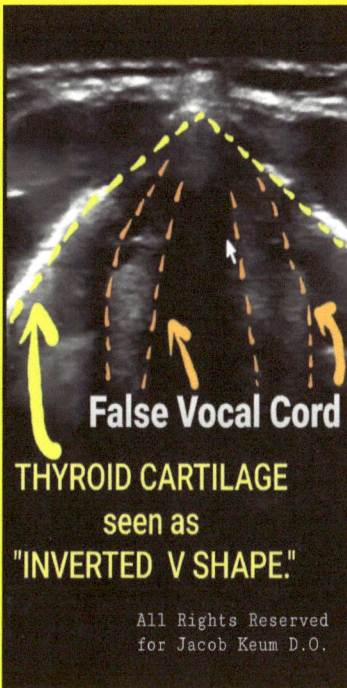

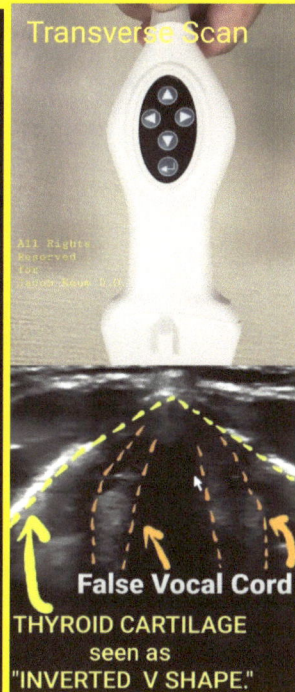

Transverse Scan

False Vocal Cord

THYROID CARTILAGE
seen as
"INVERTED V SHAPE."

False Vocal Cord

THYROID CARTILAGE
seen as
"INVERTED V SHAPE."

The **FALSE VOCAL CORDS** are located within the thyroid cartilage near the **SUPERIOR BORDER OF THE THYROID CARTILAGE**.

It is of critical importance to know that the **FALSE VOCAL CORDS** are located in the **HIGHER PLANE** than **TRUE VOCAL CORDS**. (41)

THYROID CARTILAGE
FALSE VOCAL CORDS
seen as "FROG LEGS" (by Keum)

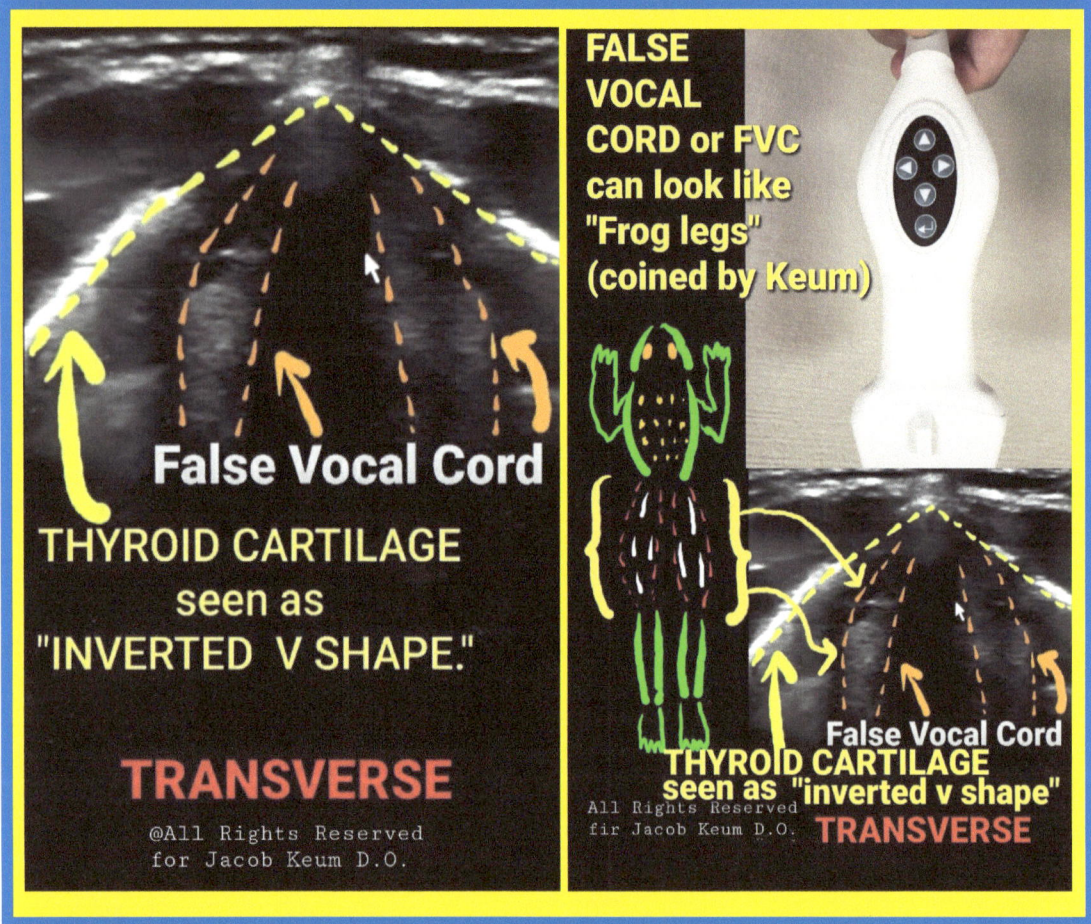

FALSE VOCAL CORD or FVC can look like "Frog legs" (coined by Keum)

False Vocal Cord

THYROID CARTILAGE seen as "INVERTED V SHAPE."

TRANSVERSE

@All Rights Reserved for Jacob Keum D.O.

False Vocal Cord

THYROID CARTILAGE seen as "inverted v shape"

All Rights Reserved fir Jacob Keum D.O.

TRANSVERSE

*FALSE VOCAL CORDS of the thyroid cartilage can resemble the shape of "FROG LEGS" particularly referring to the thigh part of FROG LEGS.

I coined this terminology because it helped me solidify my learning and make it easier to recall this structure in its sonographic view.

THYROID CARTILAGE
TRUE VOCAL CORDS SEEN AS "SWISS CHALET"(by Keum)

PROXIMAL TO SUPERIOR BORDER OF THYROID CARTILAGE, the True Vocal Cords of thyroid cartilage are seen as sharp, thin, bright structures marked in linear red ink in this scan. The True Vocal Cords can look like a smaller inverted V shape resembling the roof of a "SWISS CHALET". (Keum)

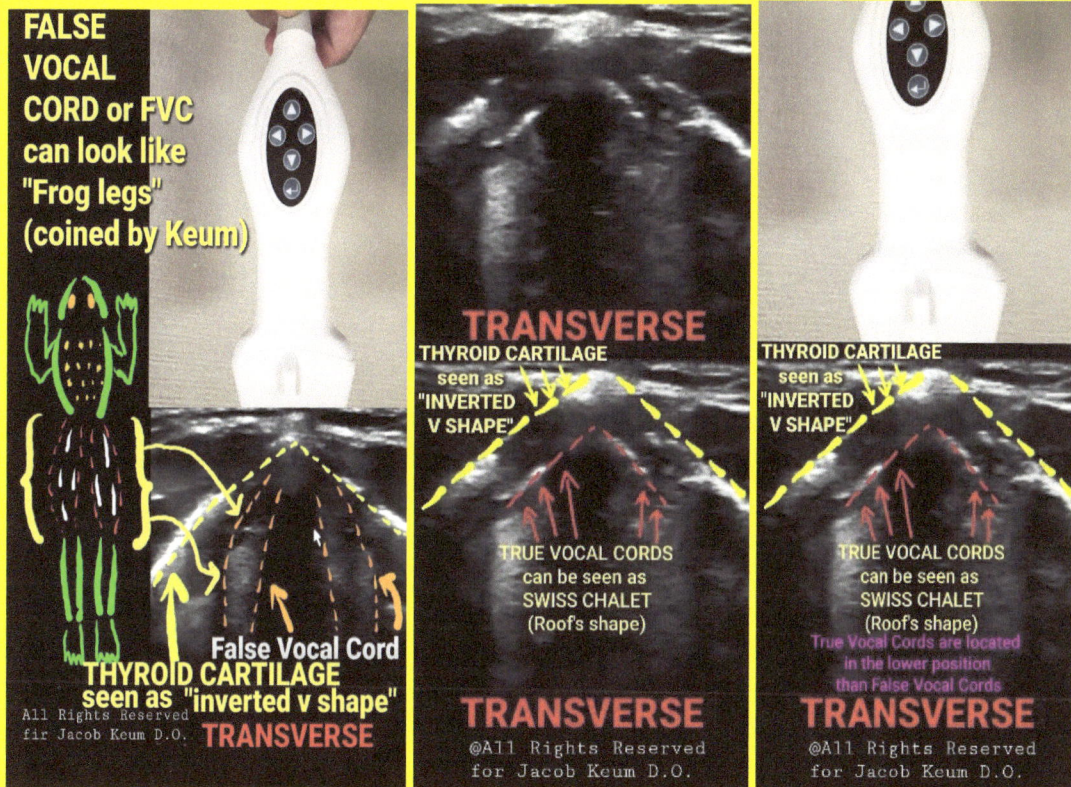

FALSE VOCAL CORD or FVC can look like "Frog legs" (coined by Keum)

False Vocal Cord
THYROID CARTILAGE seen as "inverted v shape"
TRANSVERSE

TRANSVERSE
THYROID CARTILAGE seen as "INVERTED V SHAPE"
TRUE VOCAL CORDS can be seen as SWISS CHALET (Roofs shape)
TRANSVERSE

THYROID CARTILAGE seen as "INVERTED V SHAPE"
TRUE VOCAL CORDS can be seen as SWISS CHALET (Roofs shape)
True Vocal Cords are located in the lower position than False Vocal Cords
TRANSVERSE

The False Vocal Cords looks like the thighs of "FROG LEGS" and The True Vocal Cords can look like the Roof of a "SWISS CHALET."

CRICOTHYROID MEMBRANE

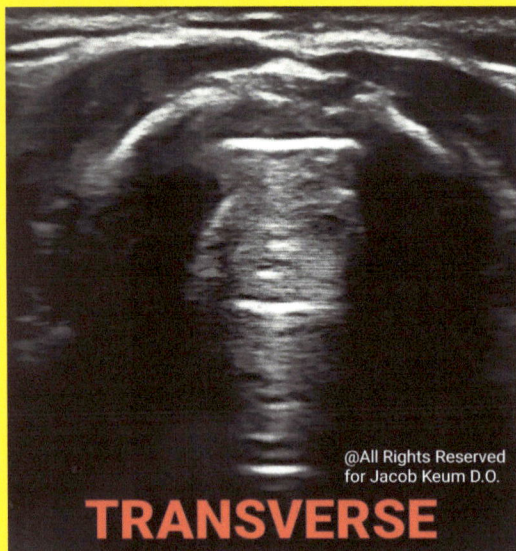

TRANSVERSE

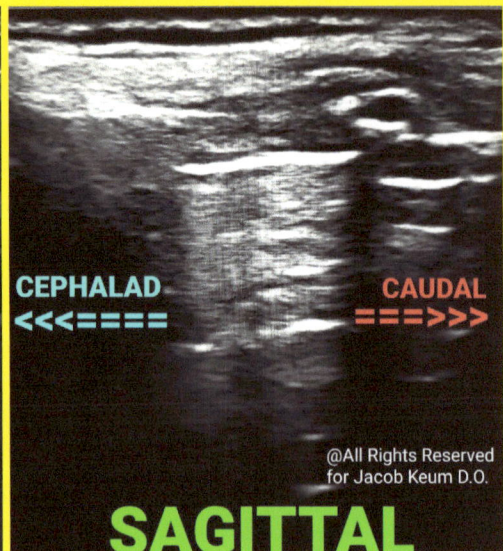

CEPHALAD
<<<====

CAUDAL
===>>>

SAGITTAL

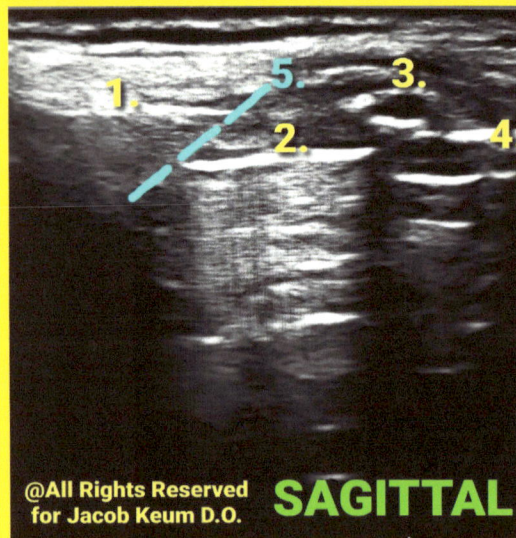

1. 5. 3.
2. 4.

SAGITTAL

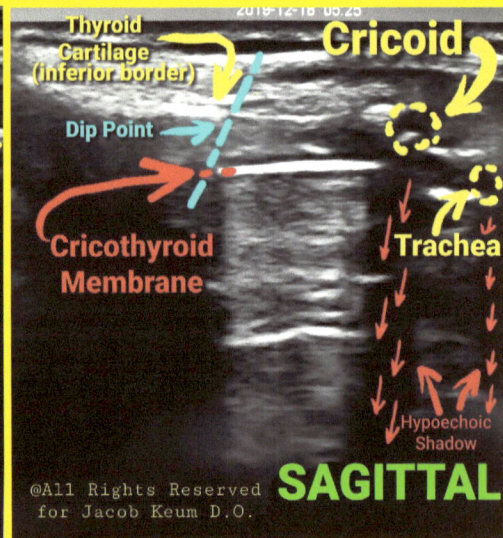

Thyroid
Cartilage
(inferior border)

Cricoid

Dip Point

Cricothyroid
Membrane

Trachea

Hypoechoic
Shadow

SAGITTAL

1. Inferior border of thyroid cartilage
2. Cricothyroid Membrane   3. Cricoid
4. Tracheal ring 1st
5. The DIP point or transition point

"DIP POINT"(keum)

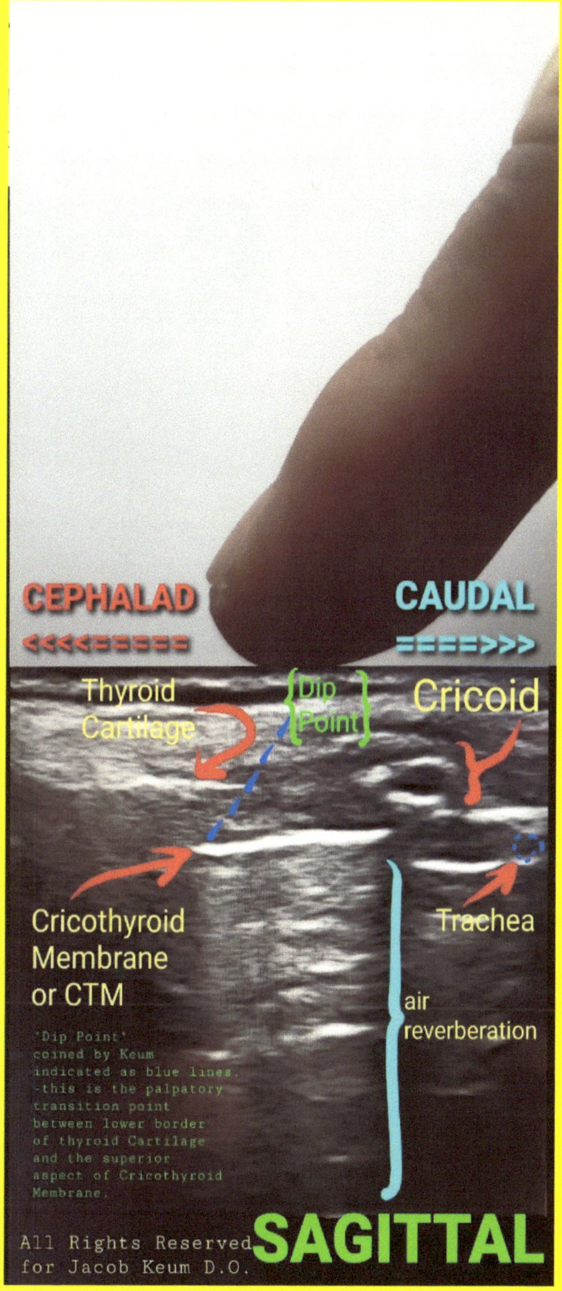

CEPHALAD
<<<<=====

CAUDAL
====>>>

Thyroid Cartilage

{Dip Point}

Cricoid

Cricothyroid Membrane or CTM

Trachea

air reverberation

'Dip Point' coined by Keum indicated as blue lines. -this is the palpatory transition point between lower border of thyroid Cartilage and the superior aspect of Cricothyroid Membrane.

SAGITTAL

"DIP POINT"

IS THE MANUAL PALPATION POINT WHICH I HAVE COINED TO DEFINE THE TRANSITIONAL ZONE WHERE THE CHANGE OR SHIFT OF PLANES OCCUR.

IT MARKS THE END OF THE INFERIOR BORDER OF THE THYROID CARTILAGE AND THE BEGINNING OF THE SUPERIOR ASPECT OF THE CRICOTHYROID MEMBRANE.

CRICOTHYROID MEMBRANE
TRANSVERSE VIEW

58

CRICOTHYROID MEMBRANE
SAGITTAL VIEW
WITH CORRELATIONS

" Two pink lines" (procedural borders) defines the area of incision

" Dip point " (the Blue line) transition from inferior border of Thyroid Cartilage to superior point of cricothyroid membrane.

@All Rights Reserved for Jacob Keum D.O.

Probe Marker Point

Thyroid Cartilage

{Dip Point}

Cricoid

Cricothyroid Membrane or CTM

Trachea

air reverberation

'Dip Point' coined by Keum indicated as blue lines. this is the palpatory transition point between lower border of thyroid Cartilage and the superior aspect of Cricothyroid Membrane

SAGITTAL

Thyroid Cartilage

{Dip Point}

Cricoid

Cricothyroid Membrane or CTM

Trachea

air reverberation

'Dip Point' coined by Keum indicated as blue lines. this is the palpatory transition point between lower border of thyroid Cartilage and the superior aspect of Cricothyroid Membrane

@All Rights Reserved for Jacob Keum D.O.

SAGITTAL

CRICOID RING

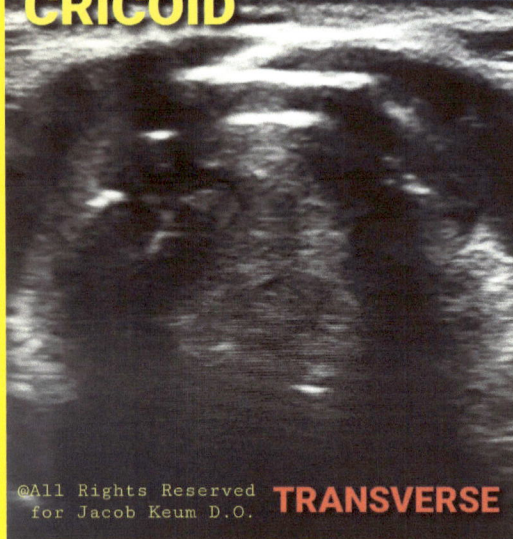

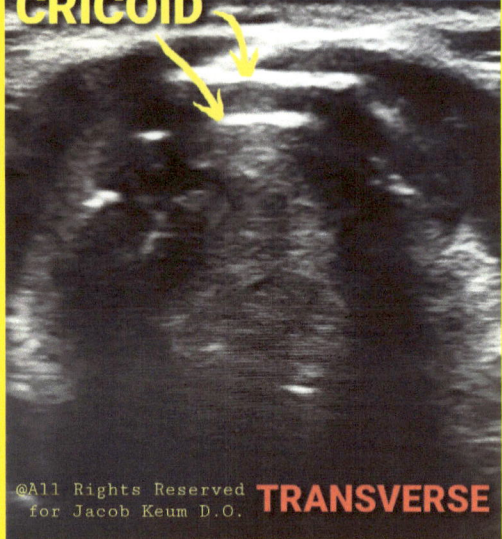

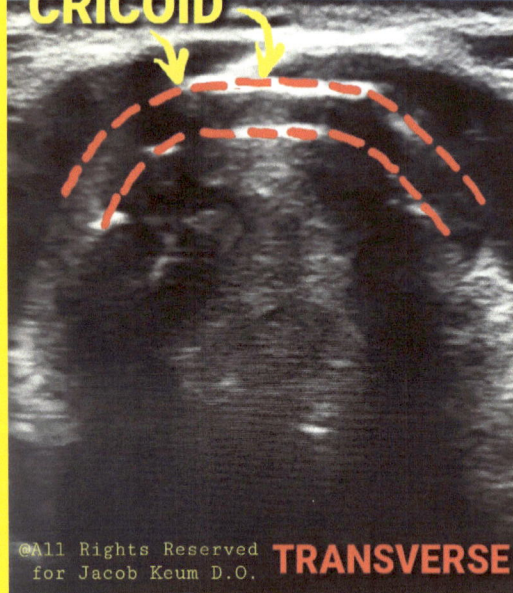

CRICOID
in TRANSVERSE Axis
May be the most difficult
to Recognize initially
but you can move caudally
the Probe starting with
the Cricothyroid Membrane
then as you reach visually
the most inferior area of
the Membrane you are able
to find it as a Hypodense
with bright linear borders
rendering a two hypoechoic
shadows.

CRICOID RING,TRACHEAL RING 1st
SAGITTAL or LATERAL VIEW

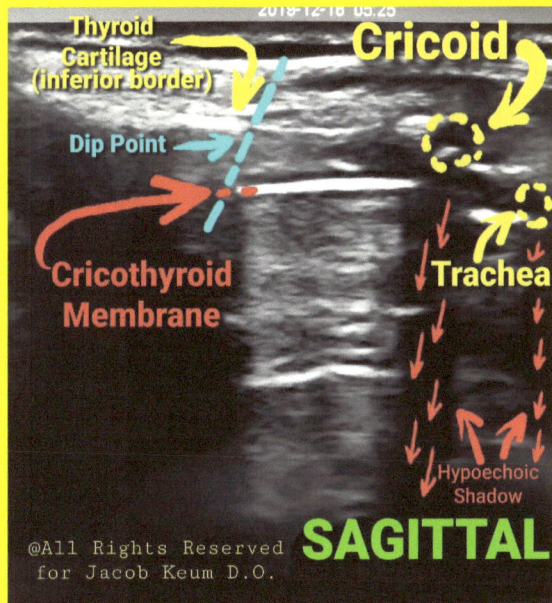

Thyroid Cartilage (inferior border)

Cricoid

Dip Point

Cricothyroid Membrane

Trachea

Hypoechoic Shadow

@All Rights Reserved for Jacob Keum D.O.

SAGITTAL

The Cricoid and the first Tracheal Ring creating a hypoechoic shadow marked by multiple red arrows.

Again, you can see the " DIP POINT " or the plane of transition from the inferior border of thyroid cartilage towards the Superior border of the CRICOTHYROID MEMBRANE indicated in TEAL COLORED LINES.

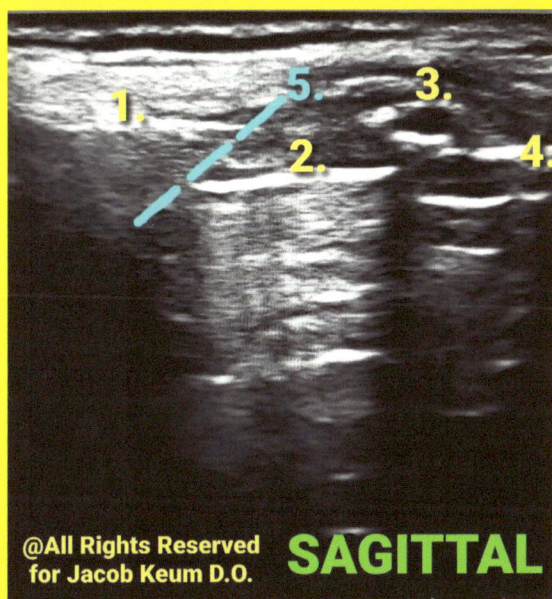

1.   5.   3.

2.   4.

@All Rights Reserved for Jacob Keum D.O.

SAGITTAL

QUICK QUIZ

1. Thyroid Cartilage (inferior border)
2. Cricothyroid Membrane.
3. Cricoid
4. Tracheal Ring 1st.
5. DIP POINT

IDENTIFY ALL THE STRUCTURES

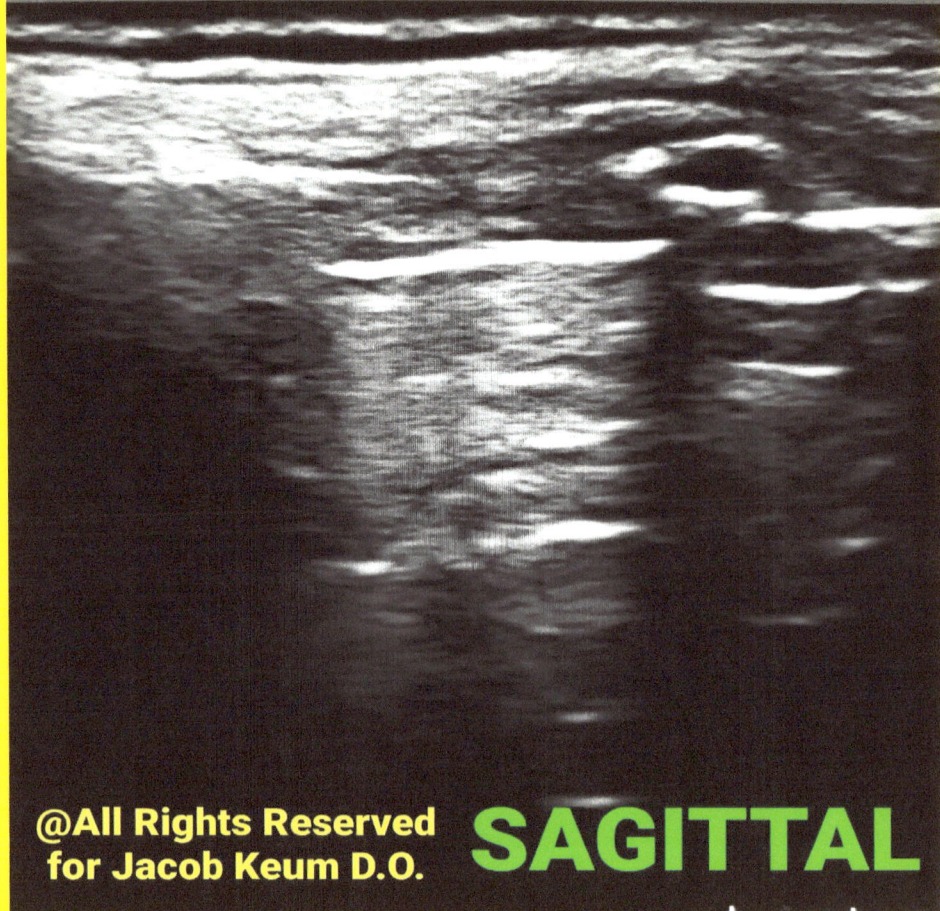

SAGITTAL

1._____

2._____

3._____

4._____

5._____

TRACHEA (<u>TRANSVERSE AXIS</u>)

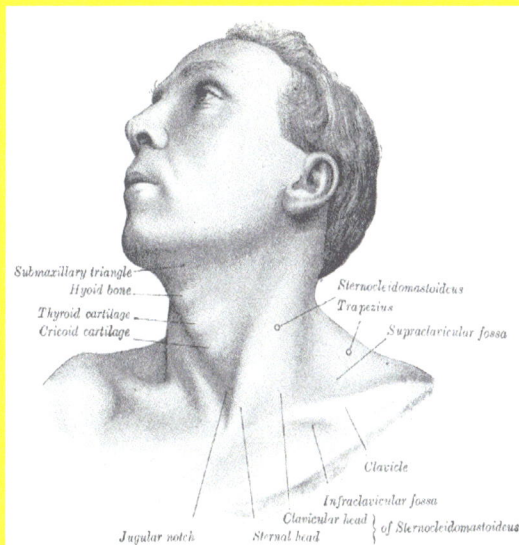

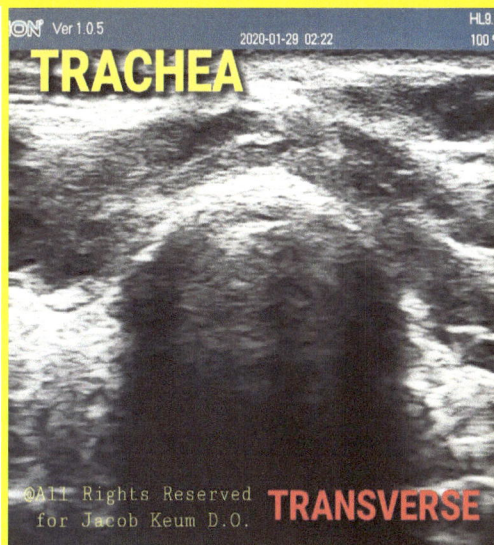

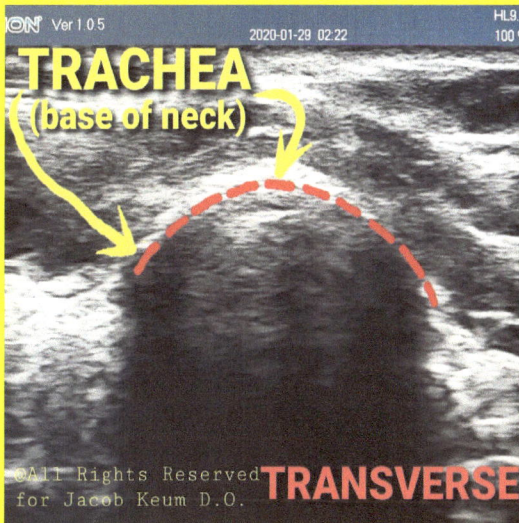

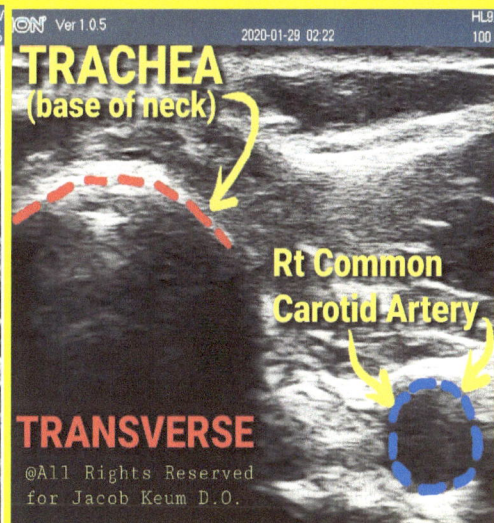

The trachea seen in the transverse axis right at the base of the neck (just superior to the jugular or sternal notch). To the right, the right common carotid artery can be identified. This vascular structure can be injured during the tracheotomy procedure. (<u>Image 1 referenced to Gray's Anatomy</u>)

Chapter 5

I have created the following cricothyroid membrane scanning protocols (they do differ from other techniques published):

> **TSTS Protocol**
> **(or Touch Scan Touch Scan Protocol)**
> **5S Protocol (5 Steps Scanning Protocol)**
> **2 Axis Confirmation**
> **2 Axis Confirmation with Procedure View (1-2-1)**
> **TC-CTM 2x Wire Protocol**
> ***Paperclip Shadow Confirmation Technique (REVIEW)**

The protocols TSTS and 5S are comprehensive scanning protocols. They scan all anatomical landmarks of interest.

The 2 Axis Confirmation, 2 Axis Confirmation with Procedure View and TC-CTM 2x wire protocol are all short-cut scanning techniques.

The practitioner should start learning the TSTS and 5S protocols first. These will serve as a solid background before moving onto the short-cut or fast techniques.

Aim to master the scanning and recognition of all important structures with accuracy as the main goal then later with improving the scanning speed.

Remember the speed is not as important as the accuracy. The scanning speed will improve with practice once you become familiarized with the scanning protocols.

TSTS PROTOCOL and Steps (by Keum)

(TSTS stands for Touch/Palpate, See/Scan then Touch/Palpate and See/Scan)

First, **Palpate** the **CHIN**. **(DON'T SCAN THE CHIN)**

Then, **Palpate** inferiorly in the **anterior aspect of the neck** and continue to:

1-**Touch/Palpate** the **Hyoid** bone (in **slightly lower plane** to **Chin** and it requires **deeper plane of palpation**)

See/Scan the **Hyoid** bone (**"Inverted Salad Bowl"**)

2-**Touch or Palpate** the **Thyroid Cartilage**

[**Superior Border of Thyroid Cartilage appears as** (**"Inverse V shaped"**)]

See/Scan The **Thyroid Cartilage**-**Superior Border** (Recognizing as the **"Inverse V shaped"** Thyroid Cartilage Superior Border is fundamental in correctly identifying the inferiorly located Cricothyroid membrane. And, remember that **the both False and True Vocal Cords are not palpable structures but visible via ultrasound scan.**)

Scan **False Vocal Cord or FVC** (**"Frog Leg" by Keum**)

Scan **True Vocal Cord or TVC** (**"Swiss Chalet" by Keum**)

3-**Touch or Palpate** the **DIP point** of the transition from one plane level to another one when moving from the **inferior border** of Thyroid Cartilage to the **superior aspect** of Cricothyroid **Membrane. (here, palpate of the Cricothyroid Membrane.)**

4-**See or Scan** the **Cricothyroid Membrane in two views**

   a. **Transverse Axis View** (**"coin slot"**) for easy recall (**keum**) Then do 90 degrees clockwise rotation of the probe while maintaining the probe in the same rotational axis point.

   b. **Sagittal Axis View** to confirm the **cricothyroid membrane** in **two views**.

TSTS PROTOCOL Scanning Steps:
Touch/Palpate Then See/Scan

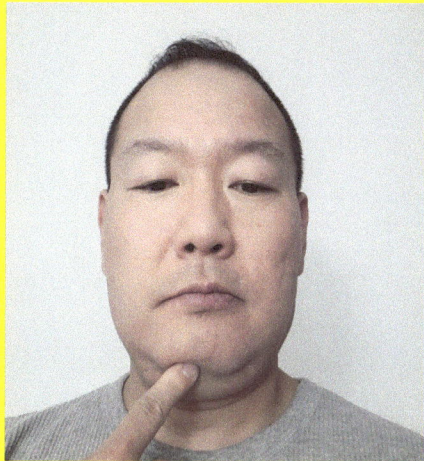

CHIN

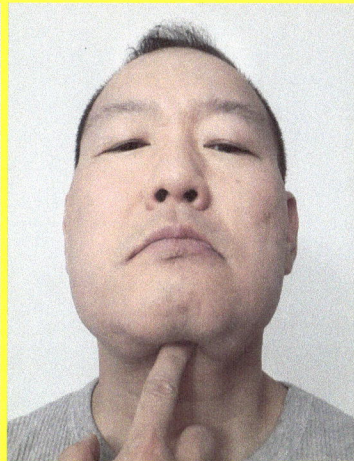

HYOID

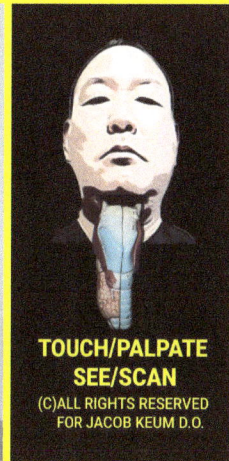

**TOUCH/PALPATE
SEE/SCAN**

(C)ALL RIGHTS RESERVED
FOR JACOB KEUM D.O.

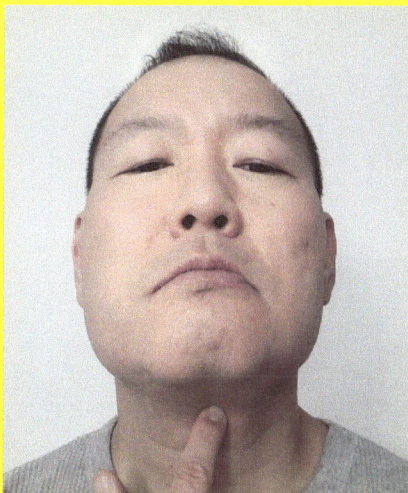

**THYROID
CARTILAGE**

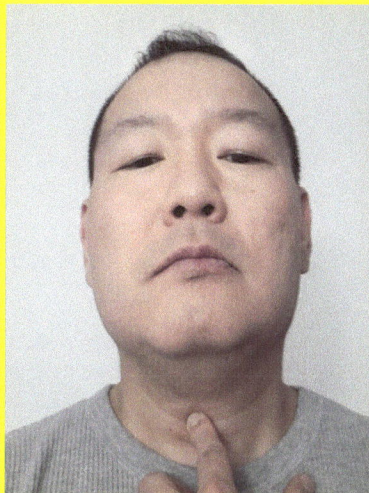

**CRICOTHYROID
MEMBRANE**

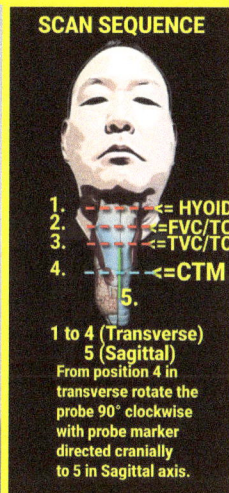

SCAN SEQUENCE

1. <= HYOID
2. <=FVC/TC
3. <=TVC/TC
4. <=CTM
5.

1 to 4 (Transverse)
5 (Sagittal)
From position 4 in
transverse rotate the
probe 90° clockwise
with probe marker
directed cranially
to 5 in Sagittal axis.

PALPATE AND SCAN SEQUENCE

(EXCEPT CHIN)

1. <<HYOID

TOUCH/PALPATE SEE/SCAN

HYOID BONE

All Rights Reserved for Jacob Keum D.O.

(C)All RIGHTS RESERVED FOR JACOB KEUM D.O.

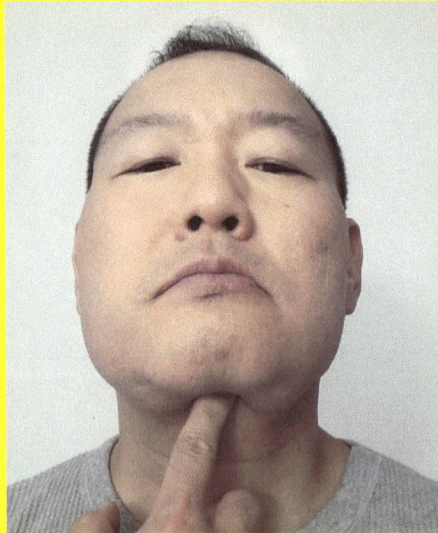

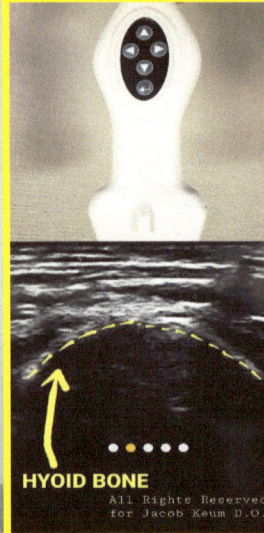

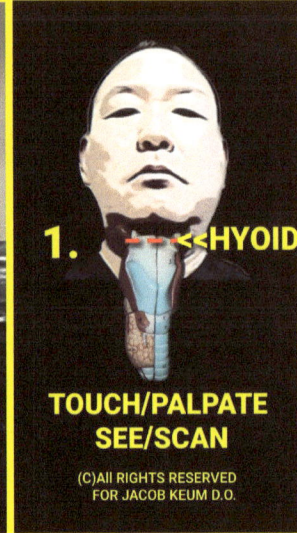

TOUCH/PALPATE THEN SEE/SCAN HYOID

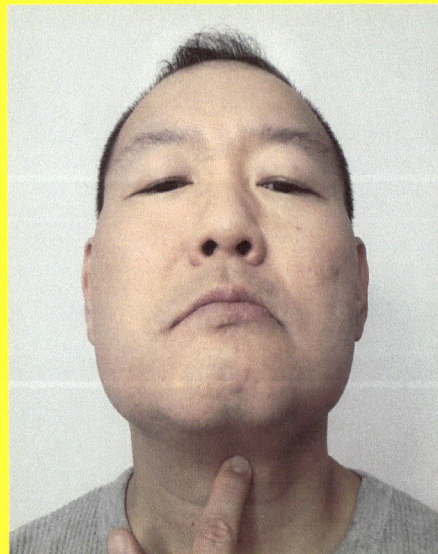

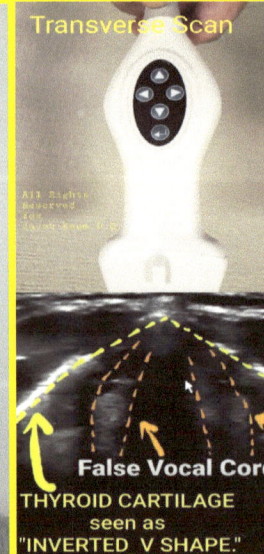

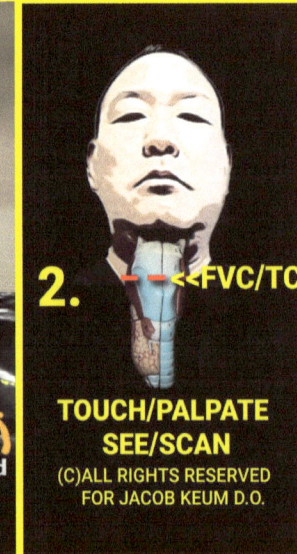

Transverse Scan

2. <<FVC/TC

TOUCH/PALPATE SEE/SCAN

False Vocal Cord

THYROID CARTILAGE seen as "INVERTED V SHAPE."

(C)ALL RIGHTS RESERVED FOR JACOB KEUM D.O.

TOUCH/PALPATE THEN SEE/SCAN THYROID CARTILAGE, FVC (At this level the FALSE VOCAL CORDS/FVC are seen FROG LEGS)

TSTS Scanning Protocol
(Continued)

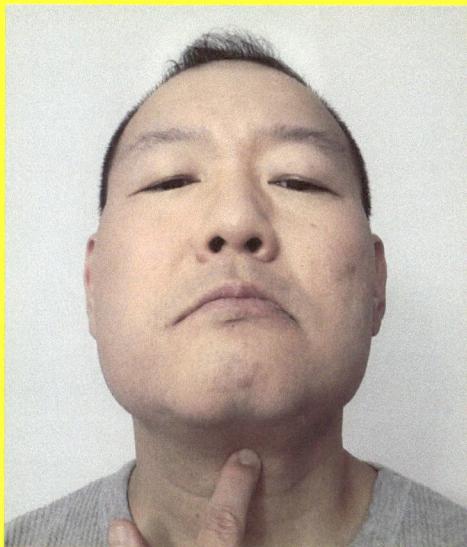

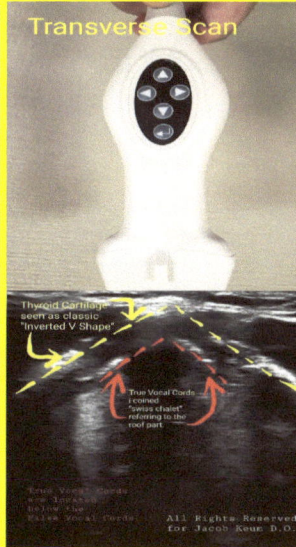

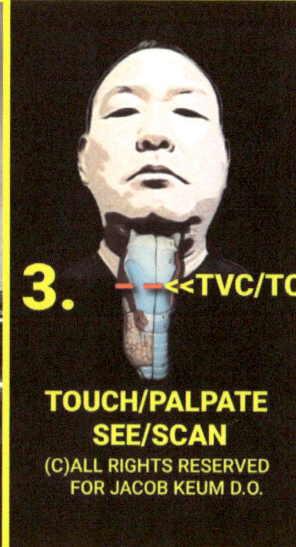

Transverse Scan

3. — — <TVC/TC

TOUCH/PALPATE SEE/SCAN
(C)ALL RIGHTS RESERVED FOR JACOB KEUM D.O.

**TOUCH/PALPATE=> SEE/SCAN THYROID CARTILAGE, TVC
(inferiorly find SWISH CHALET or TRUE VOCAL CORDS/TVC)**

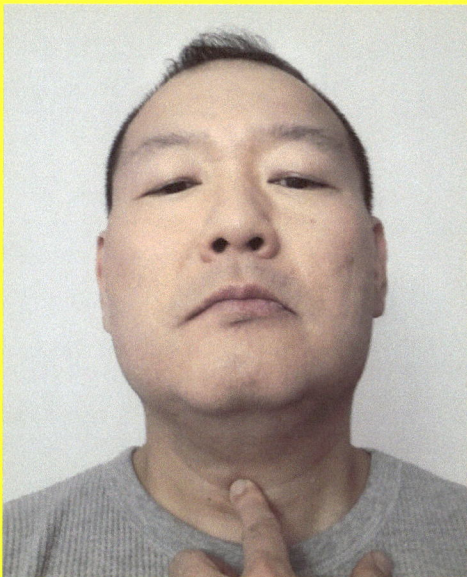

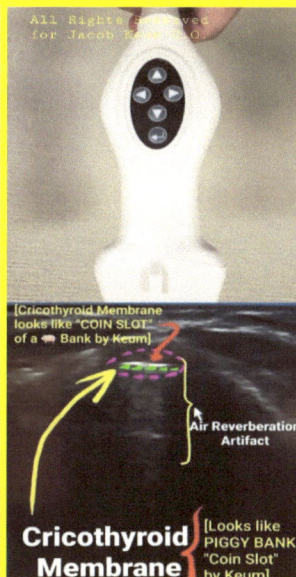

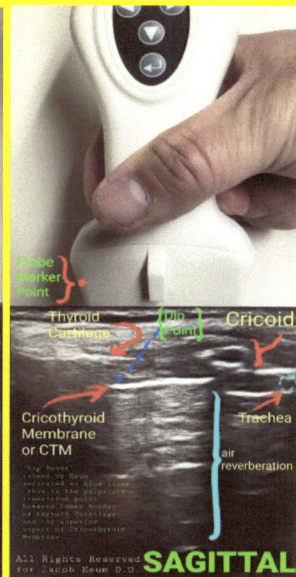

[Cricothyroid Membrane looks like "COIN SLOT" of a Bank by Keum]

Air Reverberation Artifact

Cricothyroid Membrane [Looks like PIGGY BANK "Coin Slot" by Keum]

Thyroid Cartilage Cricoid

Cricothyroid Membrane or CTM Trachea air reverberation

SAGITTAL

Palpate Cricothyroid Membrane Scan Transverse and Sagittal

TSTS SCANNING PROTOCOL cont.

Scan The Cricothyroid Membrane in 2 views
a.Transverse Axis   b. Sagittal Axis

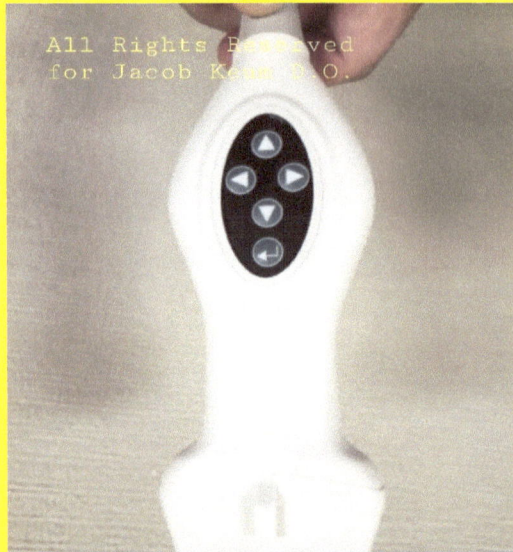

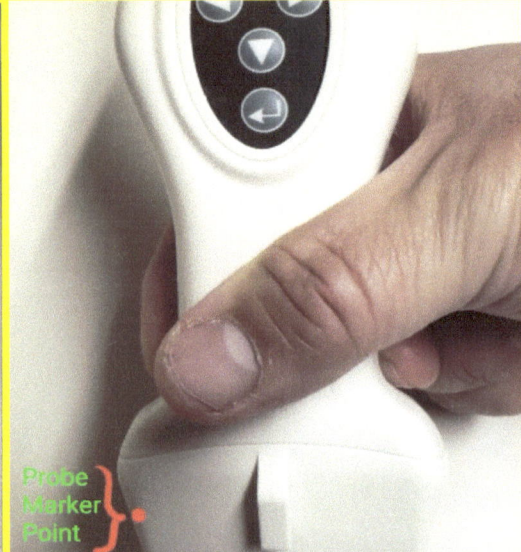

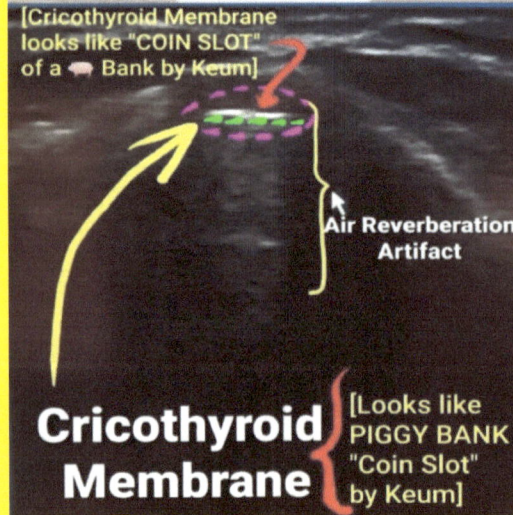

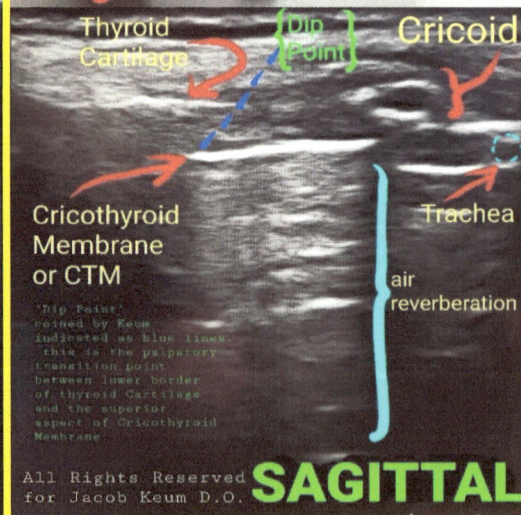

[Cricothyroid Membrane looks like "COIN SLOT" of a 🐷 Bank by Keum]

Air Reverberation Artifact

Cricothyroid Membrane [Looks like PIGGY BANK "Coin Slot" by Keum]

Probe Marker Point

Thyroid Cartilage {Dip Point} Cricoid

Cricothyroid Membrane or CTM

Trachea

air reverberation

'Dip Point' coined by Keum indicated as blue lines. this is the palpatory transition point between lower border of thyroid Cartilage and the superior aspect of Cricothyroid Membrane

SAGITTAL

The bright signal of CRICOTHYROID MEMBRANE is seen as an appearance of "COIN SLOT" of a piggy bank. (Keum)

5S SCANNING PROTOCOL STEPS:

(ONLY SCAN NO PALPATION)

5S SCANNING PROTOCOL by KEUM
Rapidly Scan 5 Views in Sequence:

1. Hyoid - " Inverted Salad Bowl".
2. Thyroid Cartilage FVC
   or False Vocal Cord. " Frog Legs"
3. Thyroid Cartilage TVC
   or True Vocal Cord.   " Swiss Chalet"
4. CTM or Cricothyroid Membrane
   in Transverse Axis
5. CTM or Cricothyroid Membrane
   in Sagital Axis

Essentially, Steps 4 and 5 are Confirmation
Steps for Cricothyroid Membrane.

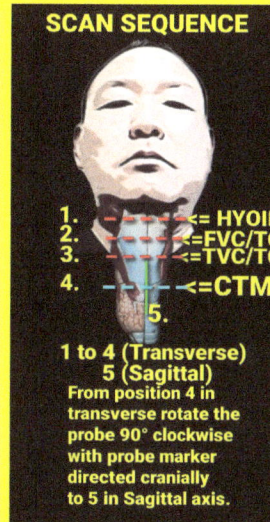

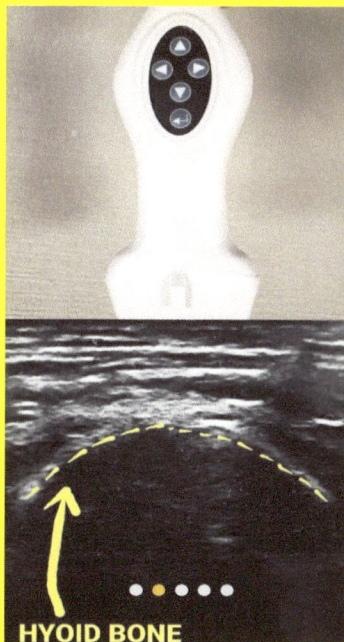

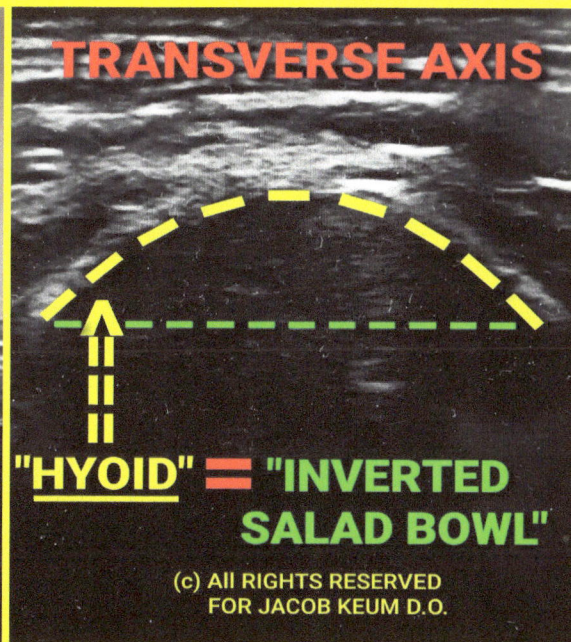

SCAN SEQUENCE

1. <= HYOID
2. <=FVC/TC
3. <=TVC/TC
4. <=CTM
5.

1 to 4 (Transverse)
  5 (Sagittal)
From position 4 in
transverse rotate the
probe 90° clockwise
with probe marker
directed cranially
to 5 in Sagittal axis.

TRANSVERSE AXIS

"HYOID" = "INVERTED SALAD BOWL"

HYOID BONE

1. Hyoid Scan

Transverse Scan

FALSE VOCAL CORD or FVC can look like "Frog legs" (coined by Keum)

False Vocal Cord

THYROID CARTILAGE seen as "INVERTED V SHAPE."

False Vocal Cord

THYROID CARTILAGE seen as "inverted v shape"

TRANSVERSE

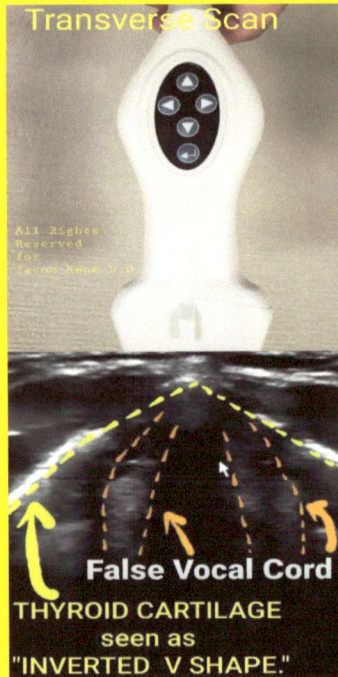

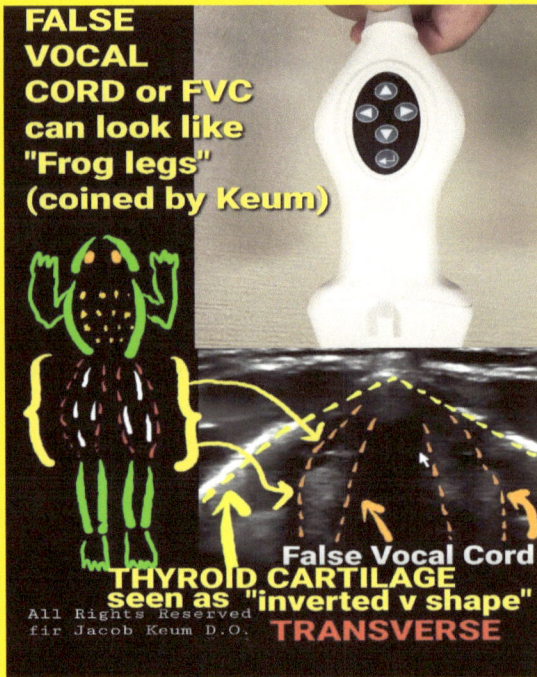

2. Thyroid Cartilage - False Vocal Cords

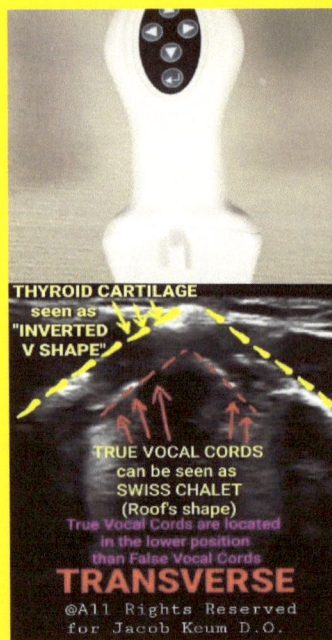

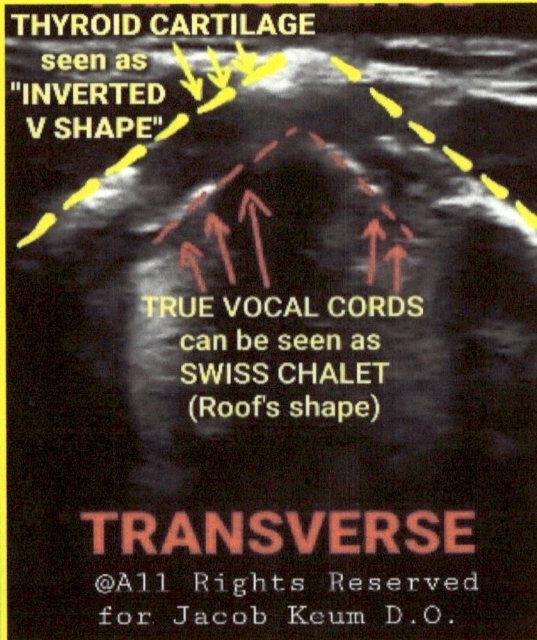

THYROID CARTILAGE seen as "INVERTED V SHAPE"

THYROID CARTILAGE seen as "INVERTED V SHAPE"

TRUE VOCAL CORDS can be seen as SWISS CHALET (Roof's shape)

TRUE VOCAL CORDS can be seen as SWISS CHALET (Roof's shape) True Vocal Cords are located in the lower position than False Vocal Cords

TRANSVERSE

TRANSVERSE

3. Thyroid Cartilage - True Vocal Cords

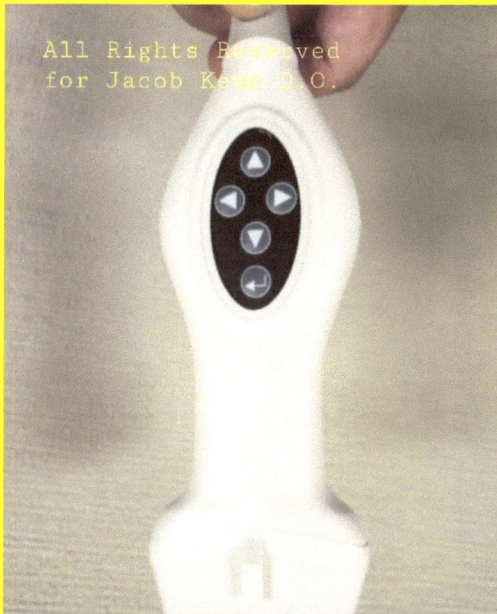

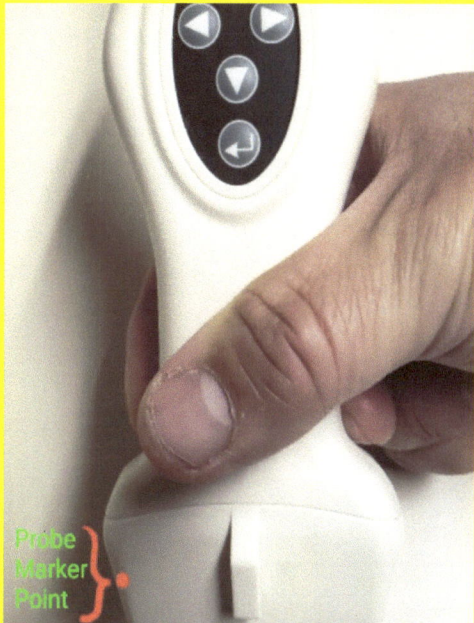

[Cricothyroid Membrane looks like "COIN SLOT" of a 🐷 Bank by Keum]

Air Reverberation Artifact

Cricothyroid Membrane { [Looks like PIGGY BANK "Coin Slot" by Keum]

Probe Marker Point

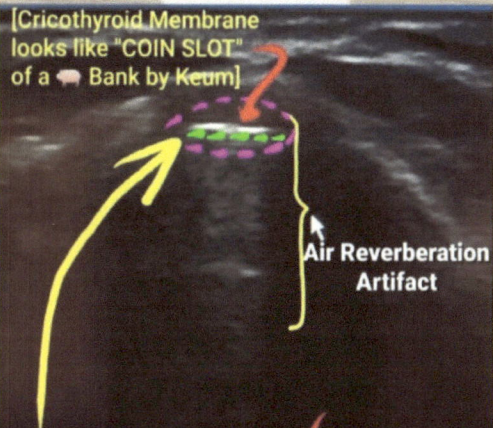

Thyroid Cartilage

[Dip Point]

Cricoid

Cricothyroid Membrane or CTM

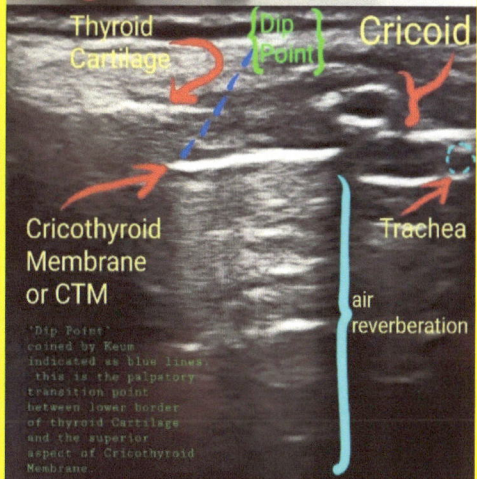

'Dip Point' coined by Keum indicated as blue lines, this is the palpatory transition point between lower border of thyroid Cartilage and the superior aspect of Cricothyroid Membrane.

Trachea

air reverberation

SAGITTAL

4.CRICOTHYROID MEMBRANE

Transverse

5.CRICOTHYROID MEMBRANE

Sagittal

2 AXIS CONFIRMATION PROTOCOL

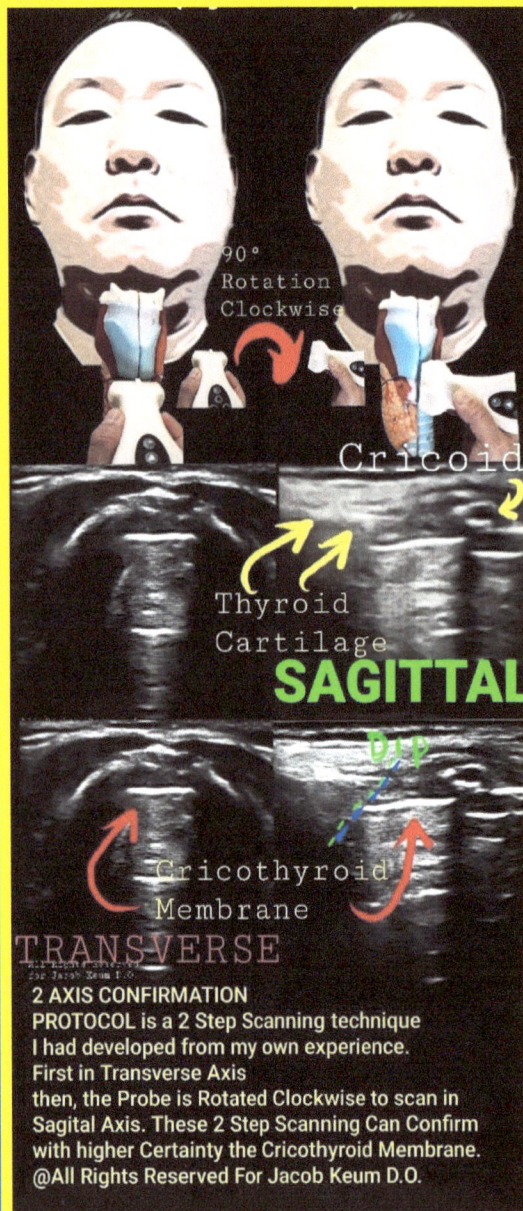

90°
Rotation
Clockwise

Cricoid

Thyroid
Cartilage

SAGITTAL

UP

Cricothyroid
Membrane

TRANSVERSE

for Jacob Keum D.O.

**2 AXIS CONFIRMATION
PROTOCOL is a 2 Step Scanning technique
I had developed from my own experience.
First in Transverse Axis
then, the Probe is Rotated Clockwise to scan in
Sagital Axis. These 2 Step Scanning Can Confirm
with higher Certainty the Cricothyroid Membrane.
@All Rights Reserved For Jacob Keum D.O.**

CRICOTHYROID MEMBRANE CONFIRMATION PROTOCOL

THE CRICOTHYROID
MEMBRANE'S EXACT
LOCATION CAN BE
CONFIRMED BY ITS
VISUALIZATION IN
2 DIFFERENT AXIS.

FIRST.

SCAN IN TRANSVERSE AXIS
TO IDENTIFY IT.

SECOND.

WE ROTATE THE PROBE 90
DEGREE CLOCKWISE WITH
PROBE MARKER CRANIALLY
DIRECTED TO IDENTIFY
THE CRICOTHYROID MEMBRANE
IN ITS SAGITTAL AXIS.

2 AXIS CONFIRMATION
ULTRASOUND VIEW

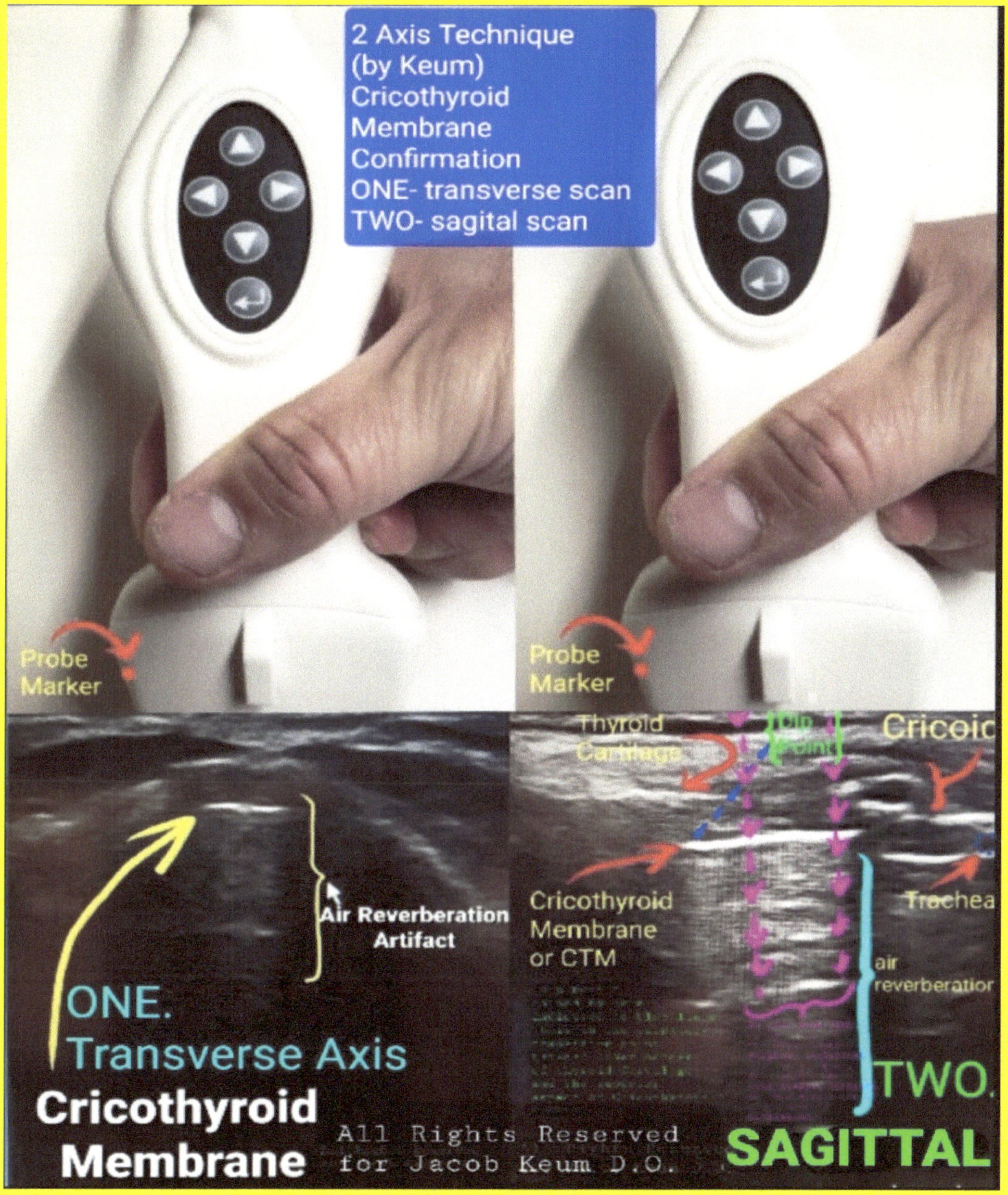

2 Axis Technique
(by Keum)
Cricothyroid
Membrane
Confirmation
ONE- transverse scan
TWO- sagital scan
Probe
Marker
Probe
Marker
Thyroid
Cartilage
Cricoid
Trachea
Air Reverberation
Artifact
Cricothyroid
Membrane
or CTM
air
reverberation
ONE.
Transverse Axis
Cricothyroid
Membrane
All Rights Reserved
for Jacob Keum D.O.
TWO.
SAGITTAL

2 Axis Confirmation with Procedure View

This Protocol requires 3 SCANNING steps:

1. TRANSVERSE AXIS VIEW
2. SAGITTAL AXIS VIEW achieved with the probe rotation counterclockwise 90 Degree from the original transverse view. The steps a and b confirms the Cricothyroid Membrane in 2 views
3. you can rotate the probe back to TRANSVERSE AXIS VIEW (step 1.) This is the PROCEDURE VIEW STEP. Using this view I find it much easier to view to do the surgical or percutaneous cricothyroidotomy procedure.

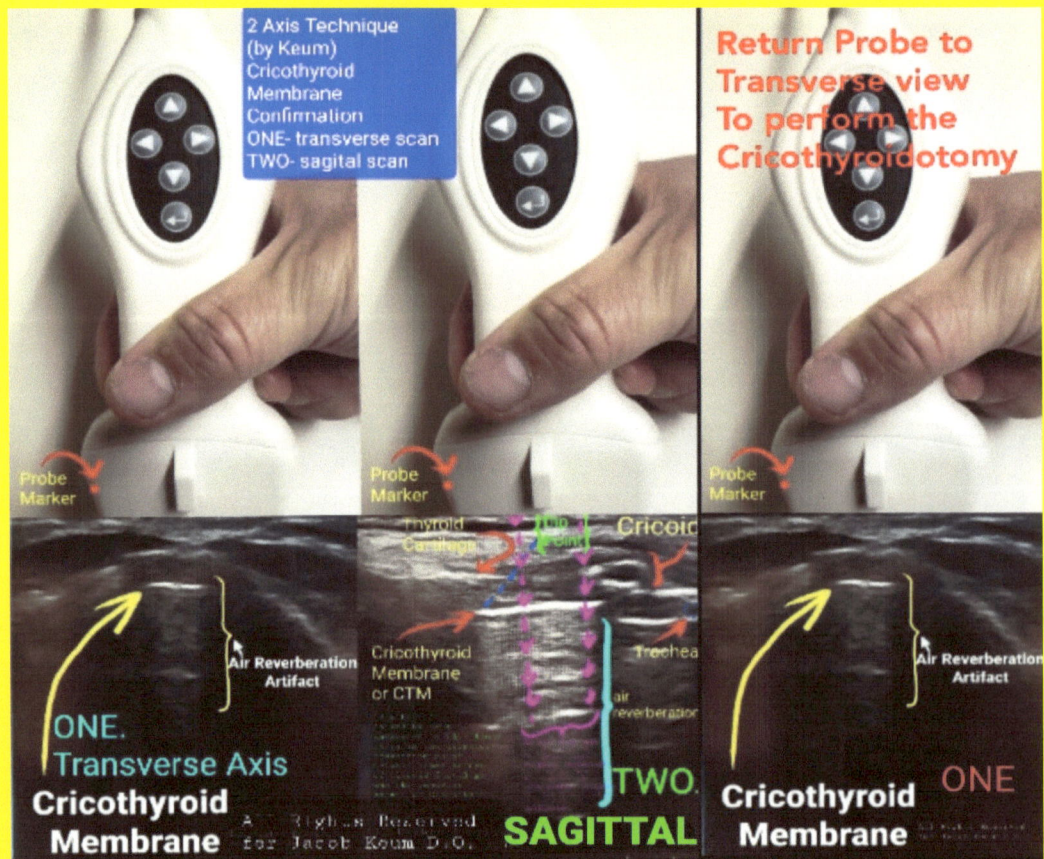

2 Axis Technique (by Keum) Cricothyroid Membrane Confirmation ONE- transverse scan TWO- sagital scan

Return Probe to Transverse view To perform the Cricothyroidotomy

Probe Marker

ONE. Transverse Axis Cricothyroid Membrane Air Reverberation Artifact

Thyroid Cartilage Cricothyroid Membrane or CTM Cricoid Trachea air reverberation TWO. SAGITTAL

Air Reverberation Artifact Cricothyroid Membrane ONE

2 Axis Confirmation
with Procedure View

(This step allows confirmation of cricothyroid membrane in 2 views then return to step 1 for procedure view.)

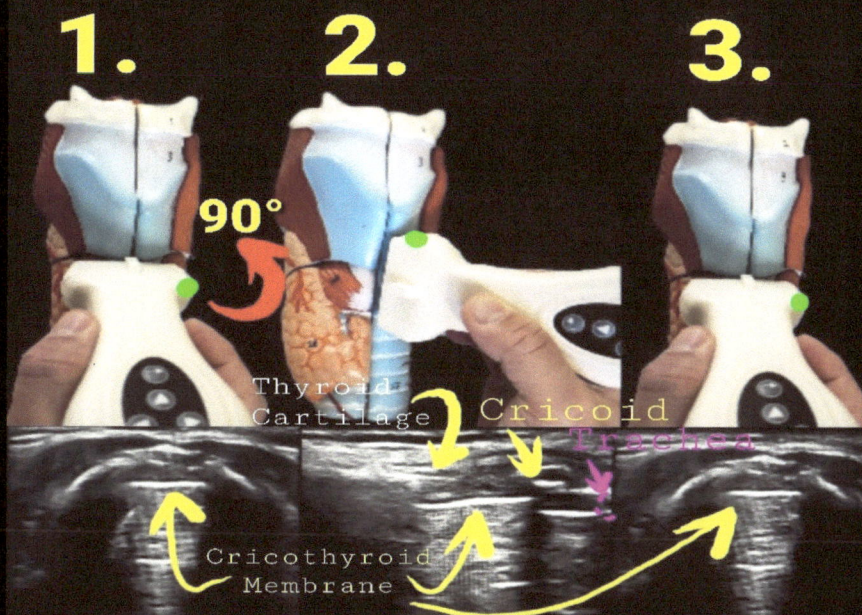

3 STEP PROCEDURE

1. 2. 3.

90°

Thyroid Cartilage

Cricoid

Trachea

Cricothyroid Membrane

TRANSVERSE **SAGITTAL** TRANSVERSE

2 Axis Confirmation with procedure step requires: scanning into following axis: Transverse->Sagital with 90° rotation counter or clockwise ->Transverse

@All Rights Reserved for Jacob Keum D.O.

PAPER CLIP SHADOW CONFIRMATION METHOD

This is a confirmation scanning method from an article published by an Italian anesthesiology group in the early 1990s. Later, this method was mentioned in other surgical airway ultrasound literature. We are not certain if the italian group was the first to propose this technique since other works do not reference the origin of this technique.

The paper clip shadow confirmation method consists of the Following:

We place a metal paperclip in its long axis between the skin and the gel impregnated probe in a transverse axis orientation. The scanned ultrasound image will show the confirmatory paperclip induced shadow.

This paperclip shadow correlates very accurately with the corresponding location in the skin correlating with the exact point of interest in the scanned images. In this case, the target is the cricothyroid membrane.

These are the steps:

First, we need a paperclip which is placed on the skin in parallel right over the cricothyroid membrane level marked in teal colored lines in transverse axis orientation.

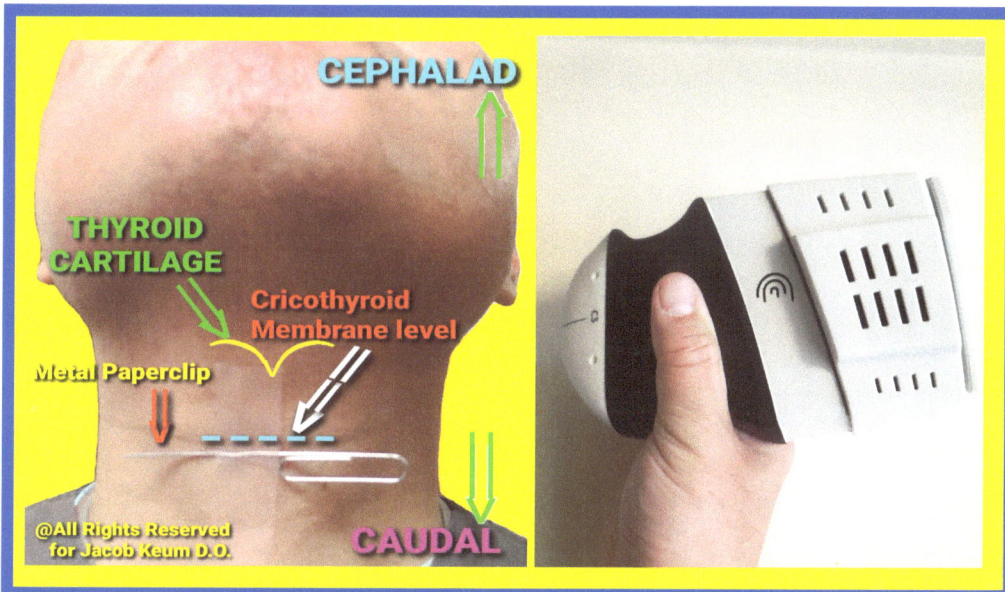

Second, place the vascular probe over the paperclip area.

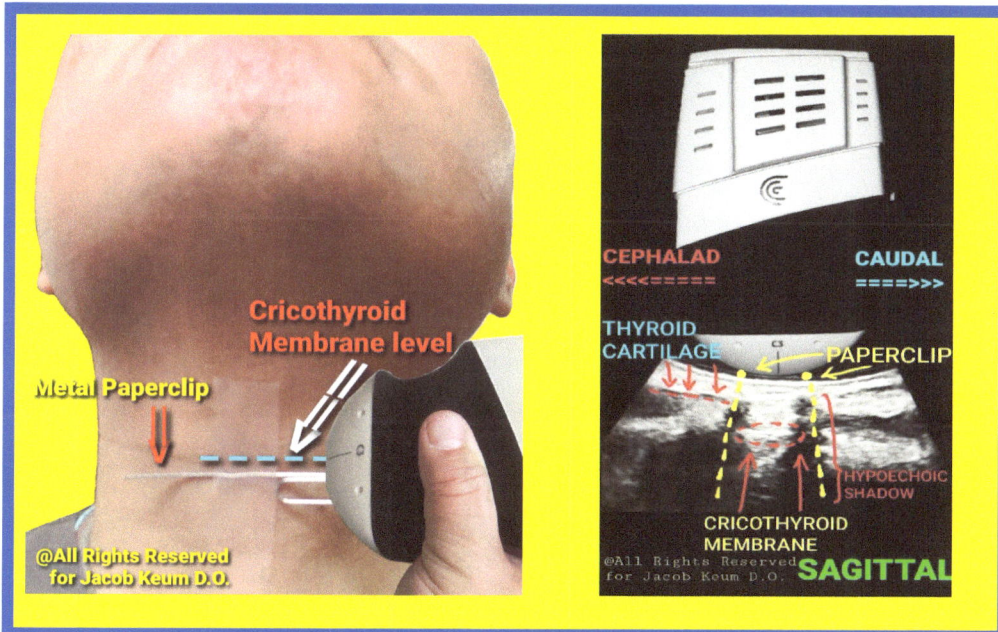

Third, view the cricothyroid membrane in the sagittal axis by moving the probe.

TWO PAPERCLIPS SCANNING PROTOCOL

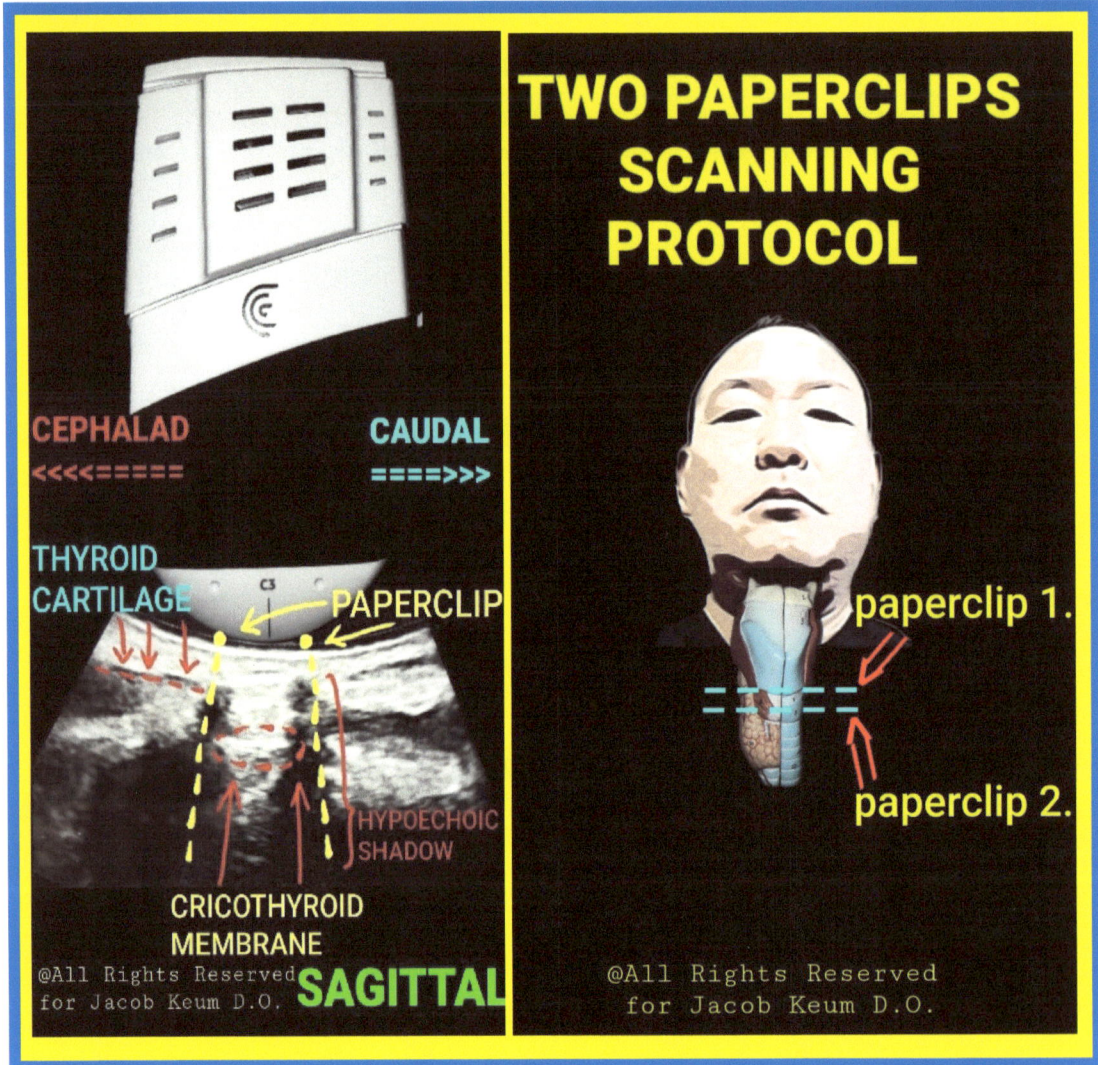

TWO PAPERCLIPS SCANNING PROTOCOL

CEPHALAD   CAUDAL

<<<<=====   ====>>>

THYROID
CARTILAGE   PAPERCLIP

HYPOECHOIC
SHADOW

CRICOTHYROID
MEMBRANE

SAGITTAL

paperclip 1.

paperclip 2.

In this particular scan, two paper clips were used: One above in the level of the superior border of the cricothyroid membrane and one below right in the level of the inferior border in parallel. Fifth, visualize the shadow artifact created by the paperclip and move it accordingly to target the cricothyroid membrane location.

Sixth step you can mark the skin with a surgical pen where the paperclip is located and proceed with the first incision of cricothyroidotomy blindly without ultrasound guidance or you can make your first incision under the ultrasound guidance.

Two types of incisions based on information from ultrasound guidance:

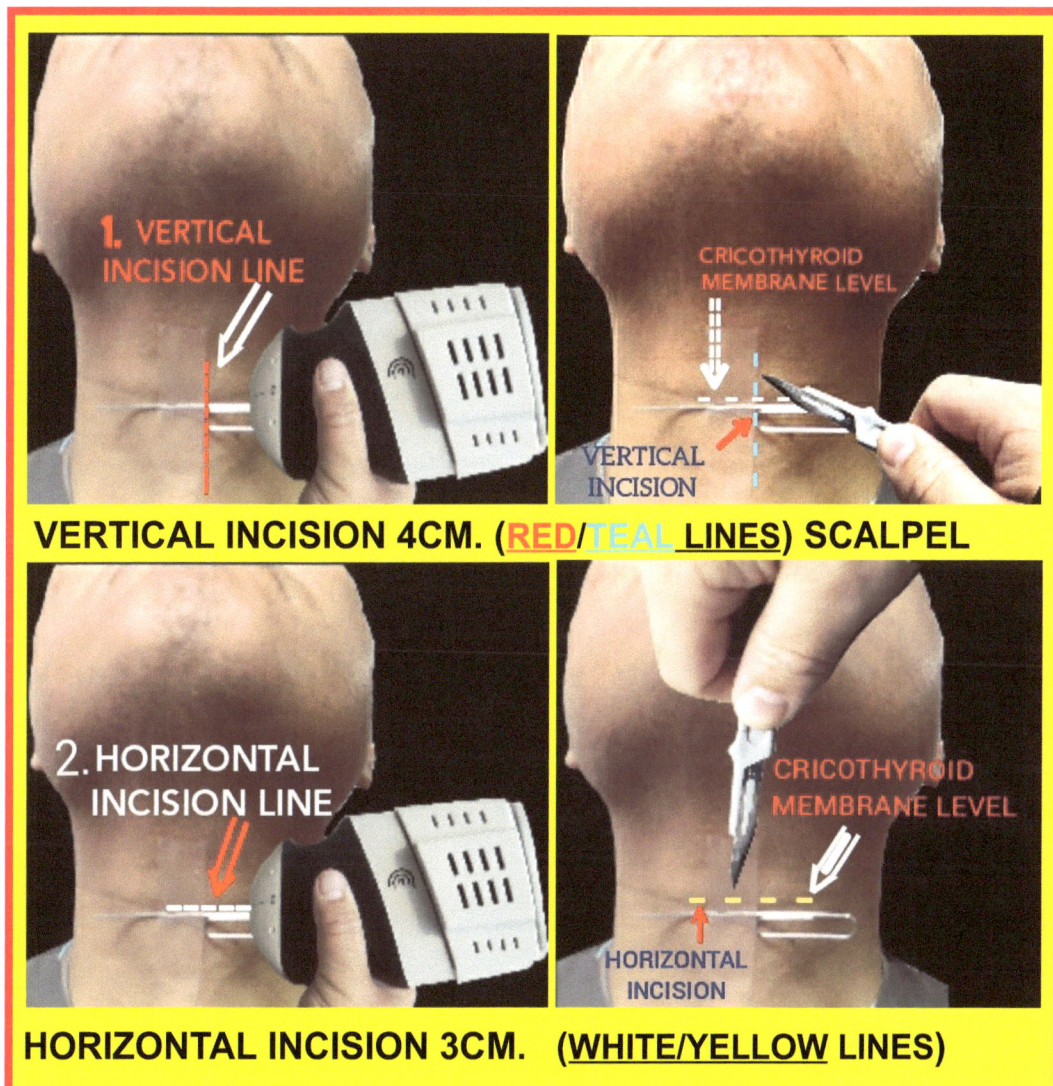

VERTICAL INCISION 4CM. (RED/TEAL LINES) SCALPEL

HORIZONTAL INCISION 3CM. (WHITE/YELLOW LINES)

The incision lines are marked with a surgical pen once you confirm with the paperclip confirmation technique. Remove the paperclip, then make the first incision of the cricothyroidotomy. In the Hennepin Regional Center's experience, the use of long vertical incision led to a decrease in complication as much as 17%.(50) Meanwhile, trauma surgeons and some emergency medicine physicians seem to prefer a horizontal incision. (27) (62)

TC-CTM 2XP Scanning Protocol

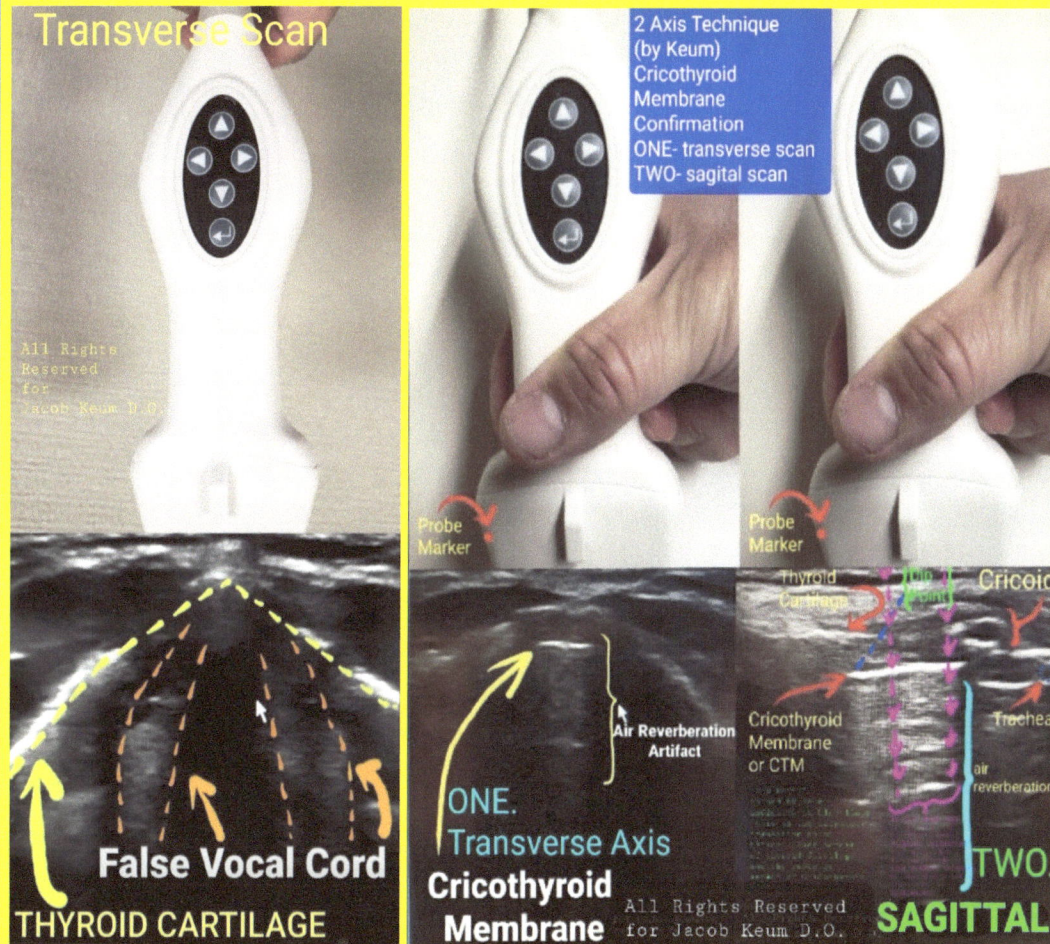

1. Scan thyroid cartilage or TC
   (identify the False Vocal Cords/Frog Legs).
2a. Scan cricothyroid membrane or CTM
   in the transverse view.
2b. Rotate the probe 90 degrees counterclockwise or
   clockwise to scan the cricothyroid membrane or CTM
   in the sagittal view.
3. Use a paperclip for correlation then mark with a skin pen.

Ex.TWO PAPER CLIPS PROTOCOL

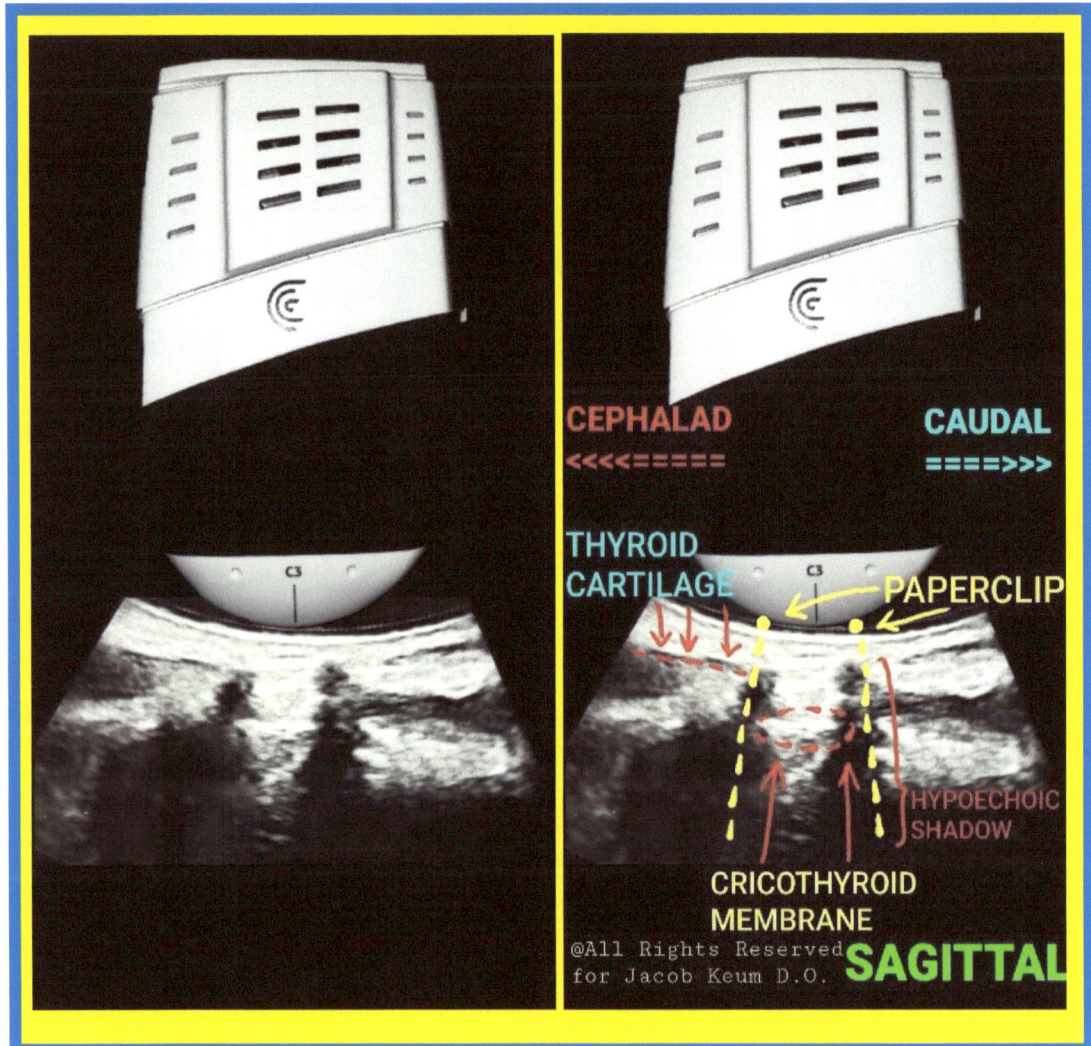

These particular scans were done with the wireless Clarius C3 ultrasound probe in vascular mode. This wireless probe is connected to an iPad, and it has been available in our Emergency Room and it is curvilinear shaped.

In my personal opinion, the Clarius C3 wireless ultrasound system is a multiscan application convex probe and it has good resolution even though a dedicated linear high frequency probes would be more ideal for this type of scanning applications. The only drawbacks of these wireless probes are two fold. It is battery powered so someone always has to make sure it is always charged. The other limiting factor would be the possible issues with connectivity or reliability of its wireless connection. I did not experience this particular problem but if your dedicated critical care or emergency department hardwired devices have access to continued outlet power supply, this may be preferable. But ultimately, the operator must decide based on his or her own preferred device for their particular scanning requirements.

Glossary and Abbreviation

Airway Surgeon	any licensed healthcare worker credentialed to perform surgical airway.
AKA	Also known as
Coin Slot	Mnemonic term for transverse view of the cricothyroid membrane
CT	Computed tomography
CTM	Cricothyroid Membrane
Dip Point	Transition point from inferior border of thyroid cartilage into superior aspect of cricothyroid membrane
D.O.	Doctor of Osteopathic Medicine
Frog Leg	Mnemonic term for false vocal cords
FVC	False vocal cord
Inverted Salad Bowl	Mnemonic term for hyoid
M.D.	Medical Doctor
MRI	Magnetic resonance imaging

Operating Surgeon	Refers to all providers performing the cricothyroidotomy procedure.
Tracheotomy, Tracheostomy	refers to same procedure a surgical procedure consists of creating an opening to the Trachea via incision or puncture.
VC	Vocal cord
Swiss Chalet	Mnemonic term for true vocal cords
TC	Thyroid cartilage
TVC	True vocal cord

Recommended Reading:

Atlas of Surgical Techniques in Trauma Demetriades 2015
Cambridge Press Chapter 2

Cook County Manual of Emergency Procedures
by Robert R. Simon, Christopher Ross, et al. | Jan 2, 2012

Atlas of Trauma/Emergency Surgical Techniques:
A Volume in the Surgical Techniques Atlas Series -
Expert Consult: Online and Print 1st Edition
by William Cioffi MD FACS (Author), Juan A. Asensio MD FACS
FCCM FRCS KM (Author), Courtney M. Townsend Jr. JR. MD
(Series Editor), B. Mark Evers MD

Ma and Mateer's Emergency Ultrasound, 3rd Edition
by O. John Ma (Author), James Mateer (Author), Robert
Reardon (Author), Scott Joing

Manual of Emergency and Critical Care Ultrasound
by Noble, Vicki E. Published by Cambridge University
Press 2nd (second) edition (2011)

Oxford American Handbook of Emergency Medicine
illustrated edition by Jeremy Brown et Al July 2008
Oxford Press pg 1072-1073

YOUTUBE VIDEO FOR CHISON Q9 OPERATIONS
https://www.youtube.com/watch?v=wb4DtdlDcg

Grey Scale Imaging Ultrasound

https://radiopaedia.org/articles/grey-scale-imaging-ultrasound?lang=us

Understanding Gain in Ultrasound

https://www.eimedical.com/blog/understanding-gain-in-ultrasound

**Principles of Color Doppler February 5th 2019
by Binder T, Altersberger M.**

https://www.123sonography.com/ebook/principles-color-doppler

References

1. Amini, R., Stolz, L.A., Gross, A. et al. Theme-based teaching of point-of-care ultrasound in undergraduate medical education. Intern Emerg Med 2015; 10: 613–618.

2. Soucy ZP, Mills LD. American Academy of Emergency Medicine position statement ultrasound should be integrated into undergraduate medical education curriculum.
J Emerg Med 2015;49:89-90.

3. Mouratev G, Howe D. Hoppmann R, et al. Teaching medical due to the much higher success rate than other target ultrasound students ultrasound to measure liver size: comparison with experienced clinicians using physical examination alone.
Teach Learn Med 2013; 25:84-8.

4. Osman A, Sum KM. Role of upper airway ultrasound in airway management. J Intensive Care 2016;4:52.

5. Garg R. Gupta A. Ultrasound: A promising tool for contemporary airway management. World J Clin Cases 2015;3:926-9.

6. Votruba J, Zemanova P, Lambert L, Vesela MM. The role of airway and endobronchial ultrasound in perioperative medicine.
Biomed Res Int 2015; 2015:754626

7. Chou HC, Tseng WP, Wang CH, et al. Tracheal rapid ultrasound exam (T.R.U.E.) for confirming endotracheal tube placement during emergency intubation. Resuscitation 2011;82:1279-84.

8. Mallin M, Curtis K, Dawson M, Ockerse P, Ahern M. Accuracy of ultrasound-guided marking of the cricothyroid membrane before simulated failed intubation. Am J Emerg Med 2014;32:61-3.

9. Kristensen MS, Teoh WH, Rudolph SS. Ultrasonographic identification of the cricothyroid membrane : best evidence, techniques, and clinical impact. Br J Anaesth 2016;117 Suppl 1:i 39-48.

10. Sustic A, Zupan Z, Antoncic I. Ultrasound-guided percutaneous dilatational tracheostomy with laryngeal mask airway control in a morbidly obese patient. J Clin Anesth 2004; 16:121-3.

11. Ezri T, Gewurtz G, Sessler DI, et al . Prediction of difficult laryngoscopy in obese patients by ultrasound quantification of anterior neck soft tissue. Anaesthesia 2003; 58:1111-4.

12. Wu J, Dong J, Ding Y, Zheng J. Role of anterior neck soft tissue quantifications by ultrasound in predicting difficult laryngoscopy. Med Sci Monit 2014; 20:2343-50.

13. Pinto J, Cordeiro L, Pereira C, Gama R. Fernandes HL, Assunção J. Predicting difficult laryngoscopy using ultrasound measurement of distance from skin to epiglottis. J Crit Care 2016; 33:26-31.

14. Chou EH, Dickman E, Tsou PY, et al. Ultrasonography for confirmation of endotracheal tube placement: A systematic review and meta-analysis. Resuscitation 2015, 90:97-103.

15. Siddiqui N, Arzola C, Friedman Z, Guerina L. You - Ten KE. Ultrasound improves cricothyrotomy success in cadavers with poorly defined neck anatomy: A randomized control trial. Anesthesiology 2015; 123:1033-41.

16. Kristensen MS, Teoh WH, Rudolph SS, et al. Structured approach to ultrasound - guided identification of the cricothyroid membrane: A randomized comparison with the palpation method in the morbidly obese. Br J Anaesth 2015; 114:1003-4.

17. Gogalniceanu P, Sheena Y, Kashef E, Purkayastha S, Paraskeva P. Is basic emergency ultrasound training feasible as part of standard undergraduate medical education? J Surg Educ 2010;67:152-6.

18. Hoppmann RA, Rao W. Bell F, et al. The evolution of an integrated ultrasound curriculum (iUSC) for medical students: 9-year experience. Crit Ultrasound J 2015;7:18.

19. Hoppmann RA , Rao W. Poston MB , et al . An integrated ultrasound Curriculum (iUSC) for medical students: 4-year experience. Crit Ultrasound J 2011;3:1-12.

20. Lamb A, Zhang J, Hung O, et al. Accuracy of identifying the cricothyroid membrane by anesthesia trainees and staff in a canadian institution. Can J Anaesth 2015; 62: 495-503

21. Bair AE, Chima R. The inaccuracy of using landmark techniques for cricothyroid membrane identification: a comparison of three techniques. Acad Emerg Med 2015; 22: 908-14

22. Brzewski M. J Ultrasound. 2017 Mar; 17(68): 41-42.

23. https://radiopaedia.org/articles/grey-scale-imaging-ultrasound? lang=us

24. https://www.eimedical.com/blog/understanding-gain-in-ultrasound

25. Enriquez JL, WU TS. An Introduction to Ultrasound Equipment and Knobology. Crit care clin 2014; 30:25-45.

26. Yadav NK, Rudingwa P, Mishra SK, Panneerselvam S. Ultrasound measurement of anterior neck soft tissue and tongue thickness to predict difficult laryngoscopy-An observational analytical study. Indian Journal of Anaesthesia 2019; 63 (8):629-34.

27. Cioffi WG, Asencio JA Atlas of Trauma/Emergency Surgical Techniques [Jurkovich GJ, Ang DN Chapter 3 Surgical Airways: Tracheostomy and Cricothyroidotomy 2014 pg 23-34]

28. Okano H, Uzawa K, Watanabe K, Motoyasu A, Tokumine J, Kawarai-Lefor A, Yorozu T. Ultrasound-Guided Identification of the Cricothyroid Membrane in a patient with a difficult airway: a case report BMC Emerg Med. 2018; 18:5.

29. Siddiqui N, Yu E, Boulis S, You-Ten KE. Ultrasound Is Superior to Palpation in Identifying the Cricothyroid Membrane in Subjects with Poorly Defined Neck Landmarks: A Randomized Clinical Trial. Anesthesiology. 2018 Dec;129(6):1132-1139.

30. Avelino, Melissa A.G. et al. First Clinical Consensus and National Recommendations on Tracheostomized Children of the Brazilian Academy of Pediatric Otorhinolaryngology (ABOPe) and Brazilian Society of Pediatrics (SBP),. *Braz. j. otorhinolaryngol.* [online]. 2017, vol.83, n.5 [cited 2020-10-14], pp.498-506

31. Jeppesen KM, Bahner DP. Teaching bedside sonography using peer Mentoring: a prospective randomized trial. J Ultrasound Med 2012; 31:455-9.

32. Griksaitis MJ, Scott MP, Finn GM. Twelve tips for teaching with Ultrasound in the undergraduate curriculum. Med Teach 2014;36:19-24.

33. You-Ten KE, Wong DT, Ye XY, Arzola C, Zand A, Siddiqui N. Practice of Ultrasound-Guided Palpation of Neck Landmarks Improves Accuracy of External Palpation of the Cricothyroid Membrane. Anesth Analg. 2018 Dec. 127(6):1377-1381

34. Alerhand S. Ultrasound for identifying the cricothyroid membrane prior to the anticipated difficult airway. Am J Emerg Med. 2018 Nov;36(11):2078-2084.

35. Walsh B, Fennessy P, Ni Mhuircheartaigh R, Snow A, McCarthy KF, McCaul CL. Accuracy of ultrasound in measurement of the pediatric cricothyroid membrane. Paediatr Anaesth. 2019 Jul;29(7):744-752.

36. Gómez-López L, Torres B, Bergé R, Aguirre O, Luis M, Sala-Blanch X. Ultrasound measurement of anatomical parameters of the upper airway in adults. Rev Esp Anestesiol Reanim. 2018 Nov;65(9):495-503.

37. Brofeldt BT et al. An Easy Cricothyrotomy Approach: The Rapid Four-step Technique Academic Emergency Medicine Nov 1996 Vol 3/NO 11

38. Foley WD, Erickson SJ. Color Doppler Flow Imaging. AJR Am J Roentgenol.1991 Jan;156(1):3-13.

39. Hwang JH et al. Principle of Ultrasound. Endosonography fourth edition 2019

40. Binder T, Altersberger M. 1.8.2.1 Principles of Color Doppler February 5th 2019 https://www.123sonography.com/ebook/principles-color-doppler

41. Moon J, Alipour F. Muscular Anatomy of the Human Ventricular Folds. Ann Otol Rhinol Laryngol. 2013 Sep; 122 (9): 561-567.

42. Boon JM, Abrahams PH, Meiring JH, Welch T. Cricothyroidotomy: A Clinical Anatomy Review. Clin. Anat. 17:478-486, 2004.

43. Hui CM, Tsui BC. Sublingual ultrasound as an assessment method for predicting difficult intubation: a pilot study. Anesthesia 2014 April volume 69, Issue 4 Pages 314-319

44. Bair AE , Chima R. The inaccuracy of using landmark techniques for cricothyroid membrane identification: a comparison of three techniques. *Acad Emerg Med* 2015; 22: 908–14

45. Walls RM. 1988. Cricothyroidotomy. Emerg Med Clin North Am.6:725-736

46. Rao S, Van Holsbeeck L, Musial JL, et al. A pilot study of Comprehensive ultrasound education at the Wayne State University School of Medicine: a pioneer year review. J Ultrasound Med 2008;27:745-9.

47. https://radiopaedia.org/articles/time-gain-compensation?lang=us,

48. https://intermountainphysician.org/intermountaincme/criticalcareecho/Documents/2014%20Content/2F-2014-Utah-Basic-Physics-Knobology-Hamlin.pdf

49. Rai Y, You-Ten E, Zasso F, De Castro C, Ye XY, Siddiqui N. The role of ultrasound in front-of-neck access for cricothyroid membrane identification: A systematic review. J Crit Care. 2020 Aug 13;60:161-168.

50. Erlandson M.J. et al. Cricothyrotomy in the emergency department Revisited. *J Emerg Med.* 1989; 7: 115-118

51. Kristensen MS, Teoh WH, Rudolph SS, Hesselfeldt R, Børglum J, Tvede MF. A randomised cross-over comparison of the transverse and longitudinal techniques for ultrasound-guided identification of the cricothyroid membrane in morbidly obese subjects. Anaesthesia. 2016 Jun;71(6):675-83.

52. Barbe N, Martin P, Pascal J, Heras C, Rouffiange P, Molliex S. Repérage de la membrane cricothyroïdienne en phase d'apprentissage: valeur ajoutée de l'échographie? [Locating the cricothyroid membrane in learning phase: value of ultrasonography?]. Ann Fr Anesth Reanim. 2014 Mar;33(3):163-6. French.

53. Basaran B, Egilmez AI, Alatas N, Yilbas AA, Sargin M. Accuracy of identifying the cricothyroid membrane in children using palpation. J Anesth. 2018 Oct; 32(5):768-773.

54. Robert r simon et al the cook county manual of emergency procedure 1st edition Chapter 1 page 49-54.

55. Demetriades et al Atlas of Surgical Techniques in trauma 2015 cambridge chapter 2

56. Frerk, C. & Mitchell, Viki & McNarry, Alistair & Mendonca, Cyprian & Bhagrath, R. & Patel, Anil & O'Sullivan, E. & Woodall, Nicholas & Ahmad, Imran. (2015). Difficult Airway Society 2015 guidelines for management of unanticipated difficult intubation in adults. British Journal of Anaesthesia. 115. 10.1093/bja/aev371.

57. Vasavada, Anita & Danaraj, Jonathan & Siegmund, Gunter. (2008). Head and neck anthropometry, vertebral geometry and neck strength in height-matched men and women. Journal of biomechanics. 41.114-21.

58. Anand, Viswanathan et al. Surgical anatomy of cricothyroid membrane with reference to airway surgeries in North Indian population: a cadaveric study. International Journal of Otorhinolaryngology and Head and Neck Surgery, [S.l.], v.4, n.5, p.1177-1181, aug. 2018.

59. Choudhary, Gagandeep.et al (2012). VALUE OF ULTRASOUND IN UNDERSTANDING LARYNGEAL ANATOMY: PICTORIAL REVIEW.

60. Arruti A, Poumayrac M. Larynx Ultrasonography:
an alternative technique in the evaluation of the aero-digestive
crossroad. Rev. Imagenol. 2010, 14(1):30-36.

61. Dover K, Howdieshell TR, Colborn GL. The dimensions and
vascular anatomy of the cricothyroid membrane: relevance
to emergent surgical airway access. Clin Anat.1996;9(5):291-5.

62. Jeremy Brown et Al Oxford American Handbook of Emergency
Medicine illustrated edition July 2008 Oxford Press
pg 1072-1073.

63. Adi, O., Sum, K.M., Ahmad, A.H. et al. Novel role of focused
airway ultrasound in early airway assessment of suspected
laryngeal trauma. Ultrasound J 12, 37 (2020).

64. Calvin A. Brown III, Sackles JC, Mick NW. The walls manual of
emergency Airway management 2018 wolters kluwer
5th edition pg 210b, 347-348, 355, 363, 412.

Index

www.ingramcontent.com/pod-product-compliance
Lightning Source LLC
Chambersburg PA
CBHW052051190326
41519CB00002BA/182